T0239356

Introduction to Horse Biology

Zoe Davies MSc (EqS)

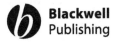

Blackwell
Publishing

Editorial Offices:
Blackwell Publishing Ltd, 9600 Garsington Road, Oxford OX4 2DQ, UK
    Tel: +44 (0)1865 776868
Blackwell Publishing Professional, 2121 State Avenue, Ames,
Iowa 50014-8300, USA
    Tel: +1 515 292 0140
Blackwell Publishing Asia Pty Ltd, 550 Swanston Street, Carlton,
Victoria 3053, Australia
    Tel: +61 (0)3 8359 1011

First published 2005 by Blackwell Publishing Ltd

Library of Congress Cataloging-in-Publication Data
Davies, Zoe.
    Introduction to horse biology / Zoe Davies.
        p. cm.
    Includes bibliographical references and index.
    ISBN 1-4051-2162-9 (pbk. : alk. paper)
    1. Horses—Anatomy.   2. Horses—Physiology.   I. Title.

    SF765.D38 2004
    636.1'0891—dc22   2004013998

ISBN 1-4051-2162-9

A catalogue record for this title is available from the British Library

Set in 10/12.5pt Palatino
by Graphicraft Limited, Hong Kong

The publisher's policy is to use permanent paper from mills that operate a
sustainable forestry policy, and which has been manufactured from pulp
processed using acid-free and elementary chlorine-free practices.
Furthermore, the publisher ensures that the text paper and cover board used
have met acceptable environmental accreditation standards.

For further information on Blackwell Publishing, visit our website:
www.blackwellpublishing.com

Contents

Preface

Study of the horse, whether at college, university or through the British Horse Society (BHS) system is becomingly increasingly popular as students search for a career in the equine sector. Equine biology is a vital subject for students wishing to study the horse and how it works, and a fundamental knowledge of this subject is essential.

Introduction to Horse Biology supplies the information required by all students of equine subjects, particularly those without a standard qualification in biology. It includes information on cells and tissues and how they function, basic microbiology and genetics. The systems of the horse are also covered extensively, with many illustrations to aid understanding. Summary points are included at the end of each chapter.

This book will be invaluable to all students of equine subjects, including First Diploma, National Diploma, National Certificate, Higher National Diploma and Advanced National Certificate, and all students studying for BHS or other equine-related examinations. It provides a good basis for students of foundation degrees without a science background, and it is ideal for serious horse owners who search for a better understanding of horses and how they function.

Zoe Davies
2004

Dedication

This book is dedicated to my husband, Ian, and daughters, Sophie and Katie, who have provided me with the time and space required to write this book and offered complete support at all times!

The Living Horse – Some Basic Principles

INTRODUCTION

To understand the way the horse works, it is important to be aware of the complex systems involved. The aim of this book is to introduce both students and horse owners to the basic structure of the horse as an animal in order that they may gain knowledge and appreciation of its capabilities and limitations. To appreciate the horse's structure and function, it is helpful to have a basic knowledge of the evolution of horses (Figure 1.1).

EVOLUTION

Most religious ideas are centred on a creator of all life. However, scientific evidence, such as the presence of fossils, tells a very different story.

Darwin's Theory of Evolution

In the 1830s, Charles Darwin (1809–1882), a naturalist from Great Britain, sailed in a ship called the Beagle, to the Galapagos Islands off the coast of South America. Here he made many observations about the animals and plants he found on the Islands, and from these he produced his Theory of Evolution.

His observations included the fact that more offspring are produced than could possibly survive, but the numbers of populations still remained fairly constant. Also, all organisms within a species showed variation, and some variations are inherited (see Chapter 14, pp. 173–82). Darwin concluded from his observations that, because more offspring were produced than survived, there must be a struggle for survival of the individual and therefore the species. The fittest and strongest of the offspring survived, and the variations, or traits, which

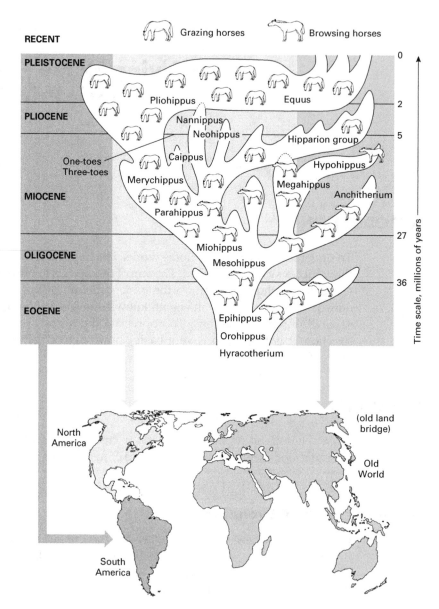

Figure 1.1 Evolution of the horse.

made them fitter and stronger were passed on in turn to *their* offspring. This process is known as *natural selection*, and it is the basis for the evolution of all species.

Natural Selection

A *species* is a group of similar organisms that breed together to produce offspring that are fertile. All horses belong to one species, *Equus caballus*, and its members share certain biological characteristics. Within a species, individuals may differ. This difference may be small or it may be big, such as the difference in height between a Shire and a Shetland, and the differences (or *variations*) may or may not be advantageous to survival.

If the environment changes over time, only the individual animals that can adapt to the new conditions will survive. These will then breed and pass on their advantageous genes to their offspring. In addition, environmental conditions, such as the number of predators, quantity of food available and occurrence of disease will also reduce the number of surviving offspring, and it will be those with advantageous variations, such as speed and immunity, that will survive. This is how natural selection works, and it is nature that 'selects' which animals survive.

Fossils

These are the remains of organisms that have died. The hard parts of the body, the skeleton for example, forms into rock and the minerals slowly infiltrate the softer parts of the body. Fossil formation takes place where there is no oxygen and it is dry and cold so that the animal does not decay but is preserved. Fossils provide great evidence for evolution. The evolution of horses is clearly shown by fossils, showing the changes in size, feet and teeth caused by changes in the environment over the years. Natural selection has resulted in the modern horse.

EVOLUTION OF HORSES

Horses may be traced back to the Eocene period, 50–60 million years ago, to a small fox-like animal known as *Hyracotherium* (also known as *Eohippus*, or 'dawn horse'). Hyracotherium was a browsing herbivore, which lived in what were then the tropical forests of North America. It is estimated to have weighed approximately 12 pounds and was 14 inches at the shoulder. Hyracotherium had four toes on the front feet and three toes on the hind feet. These were padded, similar to those of a dog. These toes and pads are now the ergots and splint bones found on the modern horse's limb.

Approximately 38 million years ago, in the Oligocene period, Hyracotherium had evolved through natural selection into *Mesohippus* then *Miohippus*, and was similar in size to a German Shepherd Dog. Due to changes in the environment, those individuals whose teeth had adapted, allowing them to browse a wider variety of plants, survived. Their front feet were now three-toed and padded, but most weight was carried on the middle toe.

In the Miocene period, approximately 27 million years ago, the defining moment in the evolution of the horse occurred. The horse's ancestors, to survive, had to move away from the tropical, swampy forests onto the plains, adapting to the new environment in a number of ways. Changes in the genetic make-up caused the head to become bigger, in order to house the longer grinding teeth, the neck to become longer, allowing the animal to reach down and graze and the position of the eyes altered to allow the animal to see the horizon whilst grazing. The limbs became longer, allowing the animal to travel at increased speeds to escape predators. These ancestors of the modern horse, known as *Parahippus* and *Merychippus*, stood most firmly on a single middle toe with side toes that were semi-functional. These animals were approximately 42 inches high (10.2 hh).

Pliohippus evolved during the Pliocene period, approximately five million years ago. The side toes were now the splint bones on either side of the cannon bones. This small slightly-built ancestor of the horse was probably the earliest prototype for *Equus caballus* (modern horse).

Equus caballus evolved during the Pleistocene period, approximately two million years ago. These animals had become well adapted to life on the open plains and were capable of great speed, having long lower limbs with an absence of muscle but a highly-muscled upper body. The foot pad of earlier ancestors is now the frog of modern horses.

Horses and other members of the family Equidae developed important social networks allowing them to live more safely in herds. These one-toed horses belonged to the genus *Equus* and these were the most recent ancestors of the horse. Figure 1.2 shows the changes to the forelimb through evolution.

Equus spread from North America to Asia, but as the glaciers retreated, approximately 10,000 years ago, land bridges between Asia and Alaska disappeared. Following this, the horse became extinct in North America, for reasons which remain unclear.

Breeds and types

Horses were domesticated at different times and places throughout the world. This has led to great variation in breeds and type, and there are now over two hundred breeds worldwide.

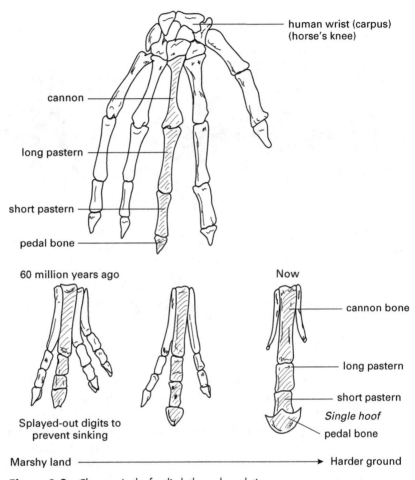

cannon

long pastern

short pastern

pedal bone

human wrist (carpus)
(horse's knee)

60 million years ago

Splayed-out digits to
prevent sinking

Now

cannon bone

long pastern

short pastern

Single hoof

pedal bone

Marshy land ———————————————————→ Harder ground

Figure 1.2 Changes in the forelimb through evolution.

Modern horses and ponies can have their origins traced back to
four basic types:

- Hotbloods – Thoroughbreds and Arabs
- Warmbloods – carriage and sports horses
- Coldbloods – heavy draught horses
- Ponies – deeper bodies and shorter legs

These types do not relate in any way to body temperature, but to
temperament and speed.

BEHAVIOUR OF THE MODERN DAY HORSE

The horse does not have the same level of intelligence as humans. In
fact, the horse's brain is small relative to its overall size (see Chapter 10,

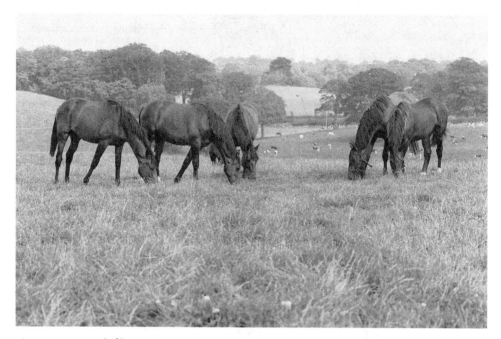

Figure 1.3 Herd of horses grazing.

p. 120), and its approach to life is based upon instincts that have evolved over many years to protect it in the wild, rather than upon thought. In the wild, the horse relied upon its highly-developed senses and a physical ability to move quickly away from the threat of attack from predators. The fight or flight response to danger seems to be highly developed in horses today, and they have the ability to move sharply and quickly away from a source of danger.

The modern-day horse retains most of the primitive instincts of its ancestors. Horses are strongly motivated to search for food and the companionship of other horses (Figure 1.3), particularly those familiar to it. This behaviour is often seen in small groups of horses or ponies in a field. When one of a close group or pair is taken away, then those left behind will often run about, whinnying frequently.

Another aspect of equine evolution that affects the horse's behaviour is the need to feed frequently. Wild horses spend most of their time grazing, eating small amounts of herbage little and often. This is known as trickle feeding and the equine gut is specially adapted to this. The horse has a tiny stomach and a large fermentation area to digest the herbage it has eaten. Whilst the horse grazes, it also walks around, helping the circulation of blood back up the leg to the heart.

It is important that the natural instincts of horses are met through correct management or horses may become depressed or 'sour' and

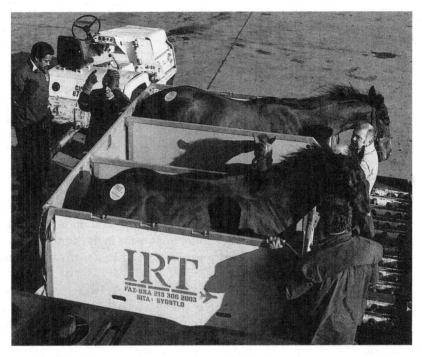

Figure 1.4 Breeding stock, including foals, may be transported abroad by plane.

uncooperative. Horses should be allowed to follow their natural instincts as much as possible. Given freedom to live as nature intended will result in healthier horses that are less likely to suffer from stress. This is particularly true of the competition horse that is often subjected to highly stressful situations including long-distance travel. Even breeding stock, including foals, may be flown abroad (Figure 1.4).

CLASSIFICATION OF LIVING ORGANISMS

Scientists have been placing organisms into groups, for the sake of comparison, for many years. As unknown organisms are found, a system of classification can help to identify them. The process of placing organisms into set groups is known as *taxonomy*.

Artificial classification

This old system used one characteristic of the organism to classify it, for example, all animals that can fly. This would include bats, birds and butterflies and obviously resulted in very different organisms in the same group.

Table 1.1   Classification of some members of the horse family.

Kingdom	Phylum	Class	Order	Family	Genus	Species
Animalia	Chordata	Mammalia	Perrisodactyla	Equidae	Equus	caballus (horse) przewalskii (Przewalskii's) asinus (donkey)

Natural classification

In the seventeenth and eighteenth centuries, two scientists, Carl Linnaeus and John Ray, developed a new, more natural, system of classification that put similar organisms in the same group. A system of smaller and smaller groups was used to classify organisms, ranging from *kingdom* to *species* (Table 1.1).

Carl Linnaeus also introduced a worldwide system known as the *Binomial System*, to help prevent confusion in naming organisms. Each organism is given two Latin names, the first being the name of the genus and the second the name of the species:

- *Equus caballus* – modern horse
- *Equus przewalskii* – Przewalskii's horse
- *Equus asinus* – donkey

The genus is always capitalised and the species is always in lower case. The name should be italicised.

Kingdom

There are five kingdoms in most modern systems:

- Animalia – all multicellular animals
- Plantae – multicellular plants that photosynthesize
- Monera – bacteria and blue-green algae
- Protista – paramecia and amoebae
- Fungi – mushrooms and toadstools

Phylum

The Kingdom Animalia is divided into 27 phyla. The horse family belongs to the phylum Chordata.

Class

Phyla and subphyla are further divided into classes:

- Amphibia – frogs and toads
- Reptilia – turtles, snakes, lizards
- Aves – birds
- Mammalia – mammals

The horse family belongs to the class Mammalia.

Order

Classes are subdivided into smaller groups called orders. The class Mammalia contains 18 different orders, including:

- Primates – humans, apes
- Perissodactyla – horses
- Artiodactyla – cows, pigs, sheep

Family

Orders and suborders are broken down into families. The horse's family is Equidae.

Genus and species

These are the final categories of the classification system. This provides the animal's scientific name, such as *Equus caballus*.

CHARACTERISTICS OF LIVING THINGS

Certain features are common to all living things, including horses. All living things, both plants and animals, have the following characteristics. They:

- **M**ove
- **R**espire – obtain energy from food
- Are **S**ensitive to stimuli
- **N**eed **N**utrition
- **E**xcrete – get rid of waste substances produced in the body
- **R**eproduce – give rise to offspring
- **G**row – get bigger until they reach adult size

This list can be remembered by the mnemonic **MRS NERG**!

Movement is obvious in a horse, but not so much in a plant. Horses have a skeleton and muscles, which enable it to move. Although most plants are rooted to the spot, their leaves and stems may be observed to move, if very slowly. When looking at plant cells under the microscope, however, they may be seen moving at some speed.

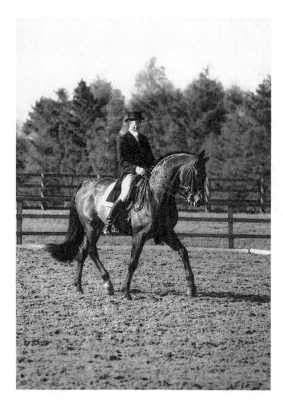

Figure 1.5 Dressage horse moving sideways.

Horses are sensitive. If you squeeze with the leg when riding, a well-trained horse should move forward as a result (Figure 1.5). The squeeze of the leg is a *stimulus* and the *response* is movement. Horses respond to heat, light, touch, sound and chemical stimuli, such as smells. Plants also respond to stimuli, but this is a very much slower response than that of animals.

Horses build up huge amounts of waste materials from all the chemical reactions going on in their cells, and these waste products need to be removed so that they do not damage the body. This process is known as excretion.

All living things need food. Horses feed on complex organic substances that are then broken down by the process of digestion to smaller, simpler particles before being absorbed into the body (Figure 1.6) – this is known as *heterotrophic* nutrition. Plants are able to make their own food from simple substances, such as carbon dioxide and water using energy provided by sunlight – this is known as *autotrophic* nutrition.

Horses must reproduce, and this involves the union of the mare and stallion, a process known as sexual reproduction. Some organisms may

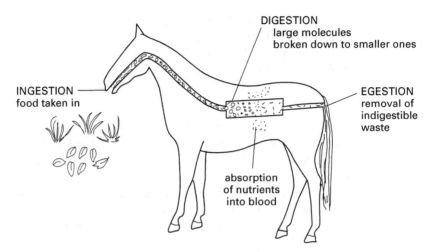

Figure 1.6 How horses digest their food.

reproduce themselves without the need for a partner and this is known as asexual reproduction.

THE HORSE'S BODY

The horse's body may be compared to a highly sophisticated machine, consisting of many different parts working together to enable the horse to live. Each of these parts has a specific function or job to do, which may be interlinked with one or several others.

Within the horse's body there are many layers of organisation and complexity:

Atoms → Molecules → Cells → Tissues → Organs → Systems

- A group of similar cells is known as a *tissue*
- A group of different tissues working together form an *organ*
- A group of organs working together create an *organ system*

For example:

Cells → Tissue → Organ → System
Nerve Nerve   Brain   Nervous System

The lowest level involves chemistry, i.e. atoms. Atoms combine to form a great range of molecules within the horse's body.

Examples of important biological molecules include:

- Water
- Carbohydrates – sugars, monosaccharides, disaccharides

- Amino acids and proteins
- Lipids (fats) – phospholipids
- Nucleic acids – DNA, RNA
- ATP – Adenosine triphosphate
- Enzymes – e.g. digestive enzymes
- Hormones – e.g. insulin, adrenalin

Cells are the smallest independent units within the body, and there are millions of them. They are specialised and perform different functions within the body, e.g. blood cells, bone cells, muscle cells, nerve cells, etc. Cells are tiny and cannot be seen by the naked eye – a microscope is required. Many cells with similar structure and function are grouped together in parts known as tissues. Examples include epithelial tissue, connective tissue, nervous tissue and muscle tissue.

Organs consist of a number of different types of tissue that together have a specific function, such as the heart, lung, liver, kidney and ovary.

Organs and tissues together work as systems required for the horse to live and survive as an individual. All these systems are required for the health of the horse.

Body systems

All the horse's body systems are interlinked in that they each have tasks to perform, but they are also dependent upon other systems.

- Respiratory system – takes air into the lungs, supplying oxygen to the body and removing waste carbon dioxide
- Cardiovascular system – heart and blood circulation; keeps the horse's body cells supplied with nutrients and oxygen and defends against disease
- Digestive system (digestive tract, pancreas, liver) – breaks down food into smaller substances that the body is able to use
- Nervous system (brain and spinal column) – control and communication network
- Endocrine system (hormones) – controls growth and internal co-ordination by chemical hormones
- Urinary system (kidneys, liver) – controls water balance
- Sensory system (eyes, ears, nose) – communicates information to the brain regarding the environment
- Reproductive system (ovaries and testes) – the smallest system, it is the only system which is different in males and females
- Musculoskeletal system – skeleton supports the body, protects major organs, provides an anchor for muscles

- Immune system – protects the horse against germs, includes white blood cells, antibodies and the lymphatic system
- Integumentary system – skin, hair, hooves, mane and tail

Movement of substances

Within the body, substances such as waste products, nutrients, hormones, etc. must move around to reach their target organs. Oxygen has to move from inhaled air and pass across the alveolar wall and then through the capillary wall deep within the lungs to reach the blood. Hormones must move from their point of manufacture to their target organs. Water, the main component of the horse's body, must move to allow distribution through the body, keeping substances (solutes) at proper concentrations to maintain the correct physiological balance. This is known as homeostasis.

Movement may occur through a variety of methods including:

- Diffusion
- Osmosis
- Active transport

Diffusion

Many substances pass in and out of cells by a process known as diffusion. Diffusion is the net movement of particles from an area of higher concentration to an area of lower concentration. There is a natural tendency for molecules to spread into all of the available space until they are evenly spread out.

Diffusion: A substance will always move from an area of high concentration to one of lower concentration, provided that there is no barrier to prevent it.

Larger molecules move at a slower rate, but the greater the difference in concentration (the concentration gradient) the faster the molecules will move. The concentration gradient can be thought of as downhill, requiring no energy to overcome. It is therefore a *passive* process. Cells take in oxygen and food for respiration from the blood and remove carbon dioxide and waste products by diffusion (Figure 1.7). The exchange of oxygen and carbon dioxide in the alveoli of the lungs also takes place by diffusion.

Facilitated diffusion

Scientists have found that some molecules are absorbed faster than others even when they have the same molecular formula, e.g. glucose

Oxygen diffuses into the cell

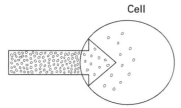

Carbon dioxide diffuses out of the cell

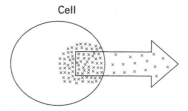

Figure 1.7   Diffusion of oxygen and carbon dioxide into and out of cells.

and fructose ($C_6H_{12}O_6$). Some particles, such as water and minerals, are also absorbed differently through the cells of the intestine. This is due to proteins within the cell membrane that provide 'channels' through which small water-soluble molecules such as glucose can pass. These proteins are known as *carrier* proteins and the process is known as *facilitated diffusion*. This process does not require energy.

Osmosis

All cells are surrounded by a cell membrane, which effectively has small holes in it. This allows some small molecules such as water to move through it. The membrane is therefore *partially permeable*. Water will actually move in both directions to attempt to even out the concentrations.

Osmosis is the process by which water moves from an area of high water concentration (weak solution) to an area of low water concentration (strong solution), through a partially-permeable or semi-permeable membrane.

If animal cells such as blood cells are immersed in water, there is less water within the blood cell than outside it, and so water will move into the cell by osmosis through the cell's partially-permeable membrane until the blood cell expands and eventually bursts. If the blood cell is placed in a more concentrated solution, water will move out of the blood cell into the surrounding solution and the cell will shrink.

Active transport

Sometimes cells need to move substances against their concentration gradient. This requires the use of energy. Some proteins within the cell membrane act as molecular pumps. These cells have an abundance of mitochondria providing ATP to power active transport. Examples of active transport are:

- Absorption of amino acids from the small intestine
- Excretion of urea from the kidney
- Exchange of sodium and potassium ions in nerve cells

Homeostasis

The horse's body must maintain a balance of many substances within it in order to work efficiently. There are many metabolic reactions constantly occurring within the cells, and enzymes control these reactions. To work properly, the correct environment of temperature, moisture, chemistry etc. is required. *Homeostasis* may be defined as the mechanism by which the horse's body maintains a constant internal environment.

Examples of homeostasis include:

- Maintaining body temperature – skin, liver and muscles
- Controlling blood sugar – pancreas, liver
- Controlling water balance – kidneys

Maintenance of body temperature is discussed in Chapter 8 and control of water balance is discussed in Chapter 5.

Control of blood sugar

The pancreas helps to maintain the level of glucose within the blood, so that there is enough for the production of energy through cellular respiration. The pancreas secretes two hormones into the blood:

- Insulin – secreted when blood sugar is too high, e.g. following high cereal starch feed
- Glucagon – secreted when blood sugar is too low, e.g. during prolonged exercise

Insulin is released as blood sugar increases. This causes the liver to take up glucose from the blood and store it as glycogen. Blood glucose levels then return to normal.

Glucagon is released as blood sugar falls, such as in prolonged exercise or starvation. Glucagon stimulates the liver to turn stored glycogen into glucose, which is then released into the blood thereby restoring glucose levels.

Summary points

- The horse has evolved over millions of years
- Changes to the overall size, limbs and head have resulted in the modern horse
- Evolution has affected the natural behaviour of horses
- Horses belong to the kingdom Animalia, phylum Chordata, class Mammalia, order Perissodactyla, family Equidae, genus *Equus*, species *caballus*
- All living things move, respire, are sensitive, need nutrition, excrete, reproduce and grow
- Cells are the smallest independent units within the horse's body
- Substances move within the body by various means, including diffusion, osmosis and active transport
- Homeostasis is vital for maintaining the balance of chemistry within the body

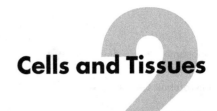

Cells and Tissues

Cells are the basic units of all life, and knowledge of the structure and function of these small independent parts is important to help in understanding how the horse's body works.

Cells are relatively independent units that are able to reproduce themselves. Cells are grouped together in tissues and the study of cells and tissues together is known as *histology*. Cells are able to carry out many functions including:

- Growth – grow and repair themselves by production of protein
- Reproduction – make new cells
- Metabolism – chemical reactions within the cell
- Excretion – removal of waste
- Movement – some cells, such as blood cells, can move around the body
- Sensation – may respond to a stimulus, for example nerve cells

When cells break down or cease to work properly, this is the beginning of disease within the horse's body.

CELL STRUCTURE

Cells are extremely small and cannot be seen by the naked eye. There are approximately 400 trillion cells within the horse's body and a typical cell would be about 20 μm wide. A light microscope, or the more powerful electron microscope, which shows more detail, is therefore required to see them.

A generalised cell and the structures within it, known as organelles, is shown in Figure 2.1.

Cell membrane

A thin layer of delicate fine membrane surrounds the outside of the cell. This membrane is made up of fat and protein threads intertwined

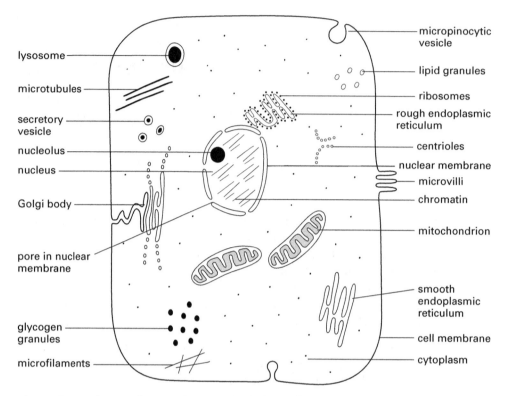

Figure 2.1   Schematic diagram of an animal cell, showing the organelles.

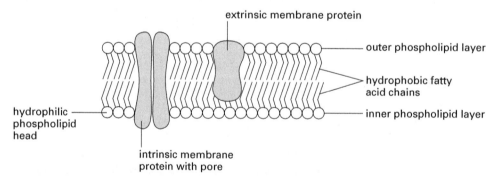

Figure 2.2   Fat and protein threads within the cell membrane.

(Figure 2.2). This membrane keeps the cytoplasm and nucleus in place within the cell but also allows the movement of some important substances into and out of the cell. The cell membrane has a structure made up of two fine layers of fat combined with a phosphate. This is known as a *phospholipid* (phospho = phosphate; lipid = fat).

Cytoplasm

The cytoplasm is a jelly-like substance consisting of approximately 70% water and additional substances such as salts, amino acids, sugars and fats. Many chemical reactions take place within the cytoplasm, which make substances, transfer energy and information and even prepare to make new cells.

The cytoplasm contains structures suspended within it, which have different functions within the cell, and these are known as cell organelles.

Cell organelles

Nucleus

This is the control centre of the cell. It controls not only all the organelles within the cytoplasm, but also cell processes such as repair, growth and reproduction. The nucleus is contained within a *nuclear membrane* and is made up of a specific nuclear material called *nucleoplasm*. This contains DNA (deoxyribonucleic acid), which holds the genetic code of the cell, and also a substance known as *chromatin*, the material from which *chromosomes* are formed.

Chromosomes are built from connected strands of DNA molecules containing genes. Genes are actually sections of the length of the DNA molecule.

Ribosomes

Ribosomes make proteins from amino acids for growth and repair of cells, using a substance called ribonucleic acid (RNA) as a template. Ribosomes are also found on the outer surface of rough endoplasmic reticulum.

Endoplasmic reticulum (ER)

The endoplasmic reticulum is a network of canals and sacs that runs throughout the cytoplasm enabling transport of substances throughout the cell. There are two types, smooth ER and rough ER, which is dotted with ribosomes on its surface.

Golgi complex (apparatus)

The Golgi complex (or apparatus) consists of stacks of closely-folded, flattened membranous sacs. It is found in all cells, but in greater amounts in cells that make and export proteins. These proteins move from the ER to the Golgi complex where they are packaged into smaller membrane-bound 'bags' known as secretory granules or vesicles. These are stored in the cell until required to be exported for use elsewhere. When needed, the proteins are then moved to the cell membrane through which they are exported.

Lysosomes

Lysosomes are one type of secretory vesicle made by the Golgi complex. They contain enzymes that break down worn out parts of the cell and engulf bacteria.

Mitochondria

These are known as the power-houses of the cell because they produce energy from respiration (Figure 2.3).

Centrioles

These are a pair of rod-like structures made up of fine tubules, which are required for cell division or *mitosis*.

Microfilaments and microtubules

Microfilaments are tiny strands of protein providing structural support and shape to the cell. Microtubules are protein structures, which can contract and are involved in movement of the cell and cell structures such as cilia.

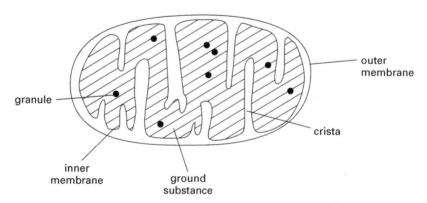

Figure 2.3   Structure of the mitochondrion.

Cell division

There are two types of cell division (Figure 2.4):

- Mitosis
- Meiosis

Mitosis

Cell division is an ongoing process throughout the horse's body. Mitosis is the multiplication of cells, allowing new cells to replace older ones, one exception being nerve cells, which are not always replaced when they die. Mitosis is the vital part of the growth process and so is faster in foals than adult horses. Mitosis takes approximately two hours to complete in an adult horse.

There are four basic stages of mitosis:

(1) *Prophase* – The centrosome divides into two centrioles, which move apart from each other on a spindle-like structure from the centrosome. The cell's nucleus contains chromatin and DNA, which shortens and thickens, turning into microscopically visible pairs of *chromosomes*. Each chromosome consists of a pair of *chromatids* joined together by a *centromere*.
(2) *Metaphase* – The nuclear membrane of the nucleus disappears and chromosomes arrange themselves at the centre of the cell attached to the *spindles* by their centromere. Towards the end of metaphase, each chromosome can be seen as two chromatids pulling apart.
(3) *Anaphase* – Pairs of chromatids divide, and identical halves of pairs move to each end of the cell. The cell membrane begins to constrict in the centre.
(4) *Telophase* – A new nuclear membrane is made around each set of chromosomes, the spindle fibres disappear and centrioles reproduce themselves. The cell membrane constricts forming two new daughter cells that are identical copies of the original parent cell, containing an identical number of chromosomes, known as the *diploid number*. The diploid number, or whole complement, of chromosomes in the horse is 64 (32 pairs).
(5) *Interphase* is the period of resting between cell divisions. DNA is copied just before mitosis begins and the parent cell increases in size.

Meiosis

Meiosis is a particular type of cell division which results in the production of a sex cell, i.e. egg or sperm. In meiosis, the daughter cells contain

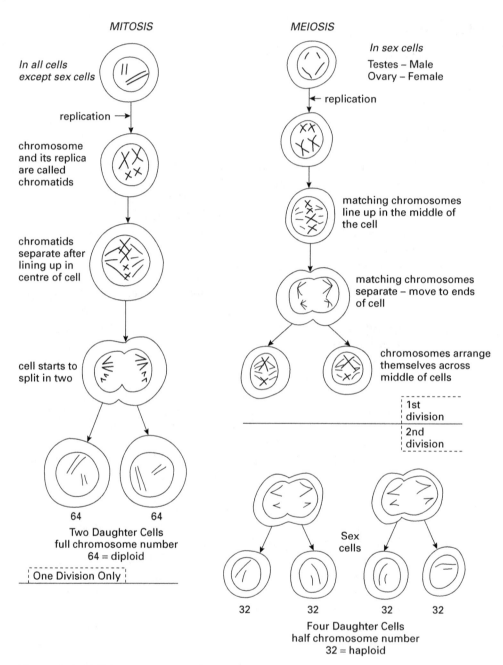

Figure 2.4 Cell division – mitosis and meiosis.

only half the number of chromosomes (known as the *haploid number*) of the parent cell, in the horse, 32. The egg or ovum contains 32 and each sperm, 32. This is so that at fertilisation, when the sperm fuses with the egg, a zygote is formed which contains the full diploid number of chromosomes. The zygote will then divide repeatedly by mitosis to form the embryo and eventually the foal.

TISSUES

Cells make up tissues, of which there are four types:

(1) Epithelial – e.g. squamous, cuboidal, columnar, compound
(2) Connective – e.g. bone, cartilage
(3) Nervous – e.g. neurones, synapses, motor end plate
(4) Muscular – e.g. cardiac, skeletal, visceral

Epithelial tissue

Epithelial tissue is more commonly known as epithelium. It may be found as simple or compound epithelium. Simple epithelium is found lining organs and vessels (such as blood vessels). Compound epithelium has more of a protective role.

Simple epithelium

Simple epithelium consists of a single layer of cells attached to a basement membrane. There are four types of simple epithelium (Figure 2.5):

(1) *Squamous* (pavement) – smooth lining for heart, blood and lymph vessels and alveoli in lungs; consists of a single layer of flattened cells attached to the basement membrane
(2) *Cuboidal* – lining of kidney tubules and glands; consists of a single layer of cube-shaped cells that can absorb and secrete substances; attached to the basement membrane
(3) *Columnar* – lines stomach, intestines and urethra; consists of a layer of taller rectangular cells attached to the basement membrane; is more resilient than other simple epithelium; some cells may secrete and some absorb mucus
(4) *Ciliated* – lines respiratory system to help remove foreign particles; consists of a single layer of mostly columnar cells, attached to the basement membrane, that have hair or finger-like projections known as cilia; works in waves to move mucus, debris and foreign material

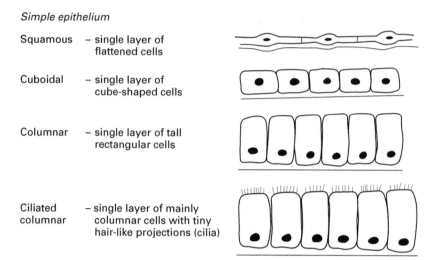

Simple epithelium

Squamous   – single layer of
                   flattened cells

Cuboidal   – single layer of
                   cube-shaped cells

Columnar   – single layer of tall
                   rectangular cells

Ciliated   – single layer of mainly
columnar   columnar cells with tiny
                   hair-like projections (cilia)

Figure 2.5 Four types of simple epithelium.

Compound epithelium

Compound epithelium consists of many layers of cells without a basement membrane. It is made up of deeper layers of columnar cells with flatter cells near and at the surface. Compound epithelium is used to protect delicate parts of the horse's body.

There are two types of compound epithelium:

(1) *Stratified* – keratinised (dry) or non-keratinised (wet); the surface layer of dry and dead cells, e.g. skin, hair, hooves. It is *keratinised* when the surface layer has dried into keratin providing a waterproof layer such as in skin; *non-keratinised* compound epithelium is wet, for example inside the horse's mouth, oesophageal lining, and conjunctiva, providing essential lubrication.
(2) *Transitional* – surface cells are pear-shaped and not flattened; found in organs needing to be waterproof and elastic, such as the bladder and ureters.

Connective tissue

These are the supporting tissues of the horse's body, i.e. muscles, ligaments, tendons and bones. They tend to have mechanical functions associated with the musculoskeletal system. Connective tissue may be solid or liquid and may have fibres present.

There are eight types of connective tissue found in the horse's body:

(1) Cartilage
(2) Bone
(3) Blood
(4) Adipose

(5) Areolar or loose
(6) Yellow elastic
(7) White fibrous
(8) Lymphoid

Cartilage

Cartilage is a tough solid tissue containing cells known as *chondrocytes*. There are three types of cartilage: *hyaline*, yellow *elastic* cartilage and white *fibrocartilage*.

Hyaline cartilage is smooth and has a blue tinge to its white colour. It is a tough cartilage, which protects and is found on articular joint surfaces and forms part of the trachea, bronchi and larynx.

Yellow elastic cartilage is made up of elastic yellow fibres running through a solid matrix. It is found in the parts of the horse's body which need to move, e.g. the horse's ear.

White fibrocartilage is extremely tough, with slight flexibility, containing white closely-packed fibres. This is a shock-absorbing cartilage and is found between joints in the horse's limbs such as the fetlock, hip and shoulder joints.

Bone

This is the hardest structure in the horse's body. Bone is a connective tissue made up of specialised cells known as *osteocytes* surrounded by a matrix of collagen fibres, strengthened by inorganic salts such as calcium and phosphate. It is made up of 25% water, 30% organic material and 45% inorganic salts. The function of bone is to support and protect the horse's body and to make cells within the bone marrow.

There are two types of bone:

(1) *Compact* – dense bone for strength
(2) *Cancellous* or spongy – cellular development and structural support

Blood

This is a fluid connective tissue, which is made up of plasma (55%) and cells (45%). The cells include red blood cells (*erythrocytes*), white blood cells (*leucocytes*) and platelets (*thrombocytes*). Blood is a transport medium, taking food and oxygen around the body and removing carbon dioxide and waste.

Adipose tissue

Adipose tissue is fatty tissue, made up of fat cells, which store fat. Adipose tissue is found under the horse's skin, giving it a smooth outline. This tissue protects and insulates, helping to maintain the horse's body temperature when it is cold. It also acts as an energy store.

Areolar or loose connective tissue

This is loose connective tissue found throughout the horse's body, supporting other tissues such as skin, blood vessels, nerves and the digestive tract. It is also found between muscles. It is semi-solid, with white fibres and yellow elastic fibres running through it. It contains *fibroblasts* and *mast cells*, which produce histamine.

Yellow elastic tissue

Yellow elastic tissue is mainly composed of elastic fibres lying in a solid matrix, and it is capable of stretch and recoil. It is found in the lungs, major arteries, stomach and bladder and other organs that need to expand.

White fibrous tissue

White fibrous tissue consists of closely-packed collagen fibres, all running in the same direction, with little elasticity. This tissue forms ligaments, tendons and the muscle fascias within the horse's musculoskeletal system.

Lymphoid tissue

Lymphoid tissue is a semi-solid tissue containing white fibres that are not aligned in any particular direction. Lymphoid tissue contains many cells, mostly *lymphocytes* (a type of white blood cell) that help to protect against disease. Lymphoid tissue forms the cells of the lymphatic system and some blood cells, and is found in the lymph nodes, thymus, the spleen, the wall of the large intestine and the glands of the small intestine.

Summary points

- Cells are the basic units of life
- There are approximately 40 trillion cells within the horse's body
- The cell contains structures within it with different functions
- There are two different types of cell division, mitosis and meiosis
- Cells are arranged in groups known as tissues

Chemistry of Life

Horses as organisms are similar to chemical factories, with hundreds of thousands of chemical reactions occurring simultaneously within the cells. The term *metabolism* describes these chemical processes of life. Some metabolic reactions build things up, a process known as *anabolism*, while others break things down, a process known as *catabolism*. Anabolic, or build-up reactions, require an *input* of energy, and these reactions are called *endothermic*. Reactions that break things down, catabolic reactions, *release* energy and are therefore known as *exothermic* reactions.

Examples of anabolic reactions are:

- Linking of glucose units to form glycogen
- Linking of amino acid units to build proteins

Respiration (see later, pp. 28–31), or the oxidation of glucose to carbon dioxide and water, is an example of a common catabolic reaction. Digestion also involves many chemical reactions, as food is broken down to simpler substances for absorption into the body.

ENZYMES

Enzymes help chemical reactions to take place. They are biological catalysts that speed up and control chemical reactions within the horse's body. Without enzymes to speed things up, life could not exist. An example of the importance of enzymes is catalase. This enzyme breaks down poisonous hydrogen peroxide that is formed within the liver to harmless water and oxygen. One molecule of catalase can break down six million molecules of hydrogen peroxide in around one minute!

Enzymes are made within the cells and may be used inside the cell (*intracellular* enzymes) or transported outside for use elsewhere (*extracellular* enzymes). Examples of extracellular enzymes are those enzymes associated with digestion in the gut.

Characteristics of enzymes

The normal activity of enzymes will depend upon the environment and abnormal conditions will reduce enzyme activity. For example, enzymes will have an *optimum*, or ideal, temperature at which they function. Some enzymes work better if other substances are also present. An example of this is lipase, which digests fat in the stomach. This works more effectively when emulsifying agents that break up the fat into smaller droplets are present. Pepsin from the stomach, which breaks down protein, works better in the acid environment of the stomach.

All enzymes have certain characteristics in common:

- All enzymes are proteins
- Control a particular chemical reaction
- Reusable
- Inactivated or otherwise damaged by heat
- Sensitive to acid and/or alkali
- Mostly prefer neutral pH

An example of an enzyme-controlled reaction is the break down of maltose to glucose:

Maltase   (enzyme)

Maltose ◄------------------► Glucose

(substrate)   (product)

Maltase is the enzyme catalysing this reaction, acting upon maltose (*substrate*) and resulting in glucose (*product*). This reaction is reversible, in that maltase may also convert glucose to maltose if there is a high concentration of glucose.

Figure 3.1 demonstrates how enzymes work.

RESPIRATION

All animals need energy for biological functions including growth, work, pregnancy and just moving about and living. Energy is derived from the breakdown of food to carbon dioxide and water, a process known as *respiration*, or *cellular respiration*. This normally occurs in the presence of oxygen, which horses breathe in. The term *respiration* may lead to confusion. It is often thought of as breathing only but it is also one of the seven characteristics of life. Respiration in the metabolic sense, which refers to oxidation of food to provide energy, is also known as *cellular respiration* and should not be confused with breathing. Comparisons of the energy released by the breakdown of different food types are shown in Table 3.1.

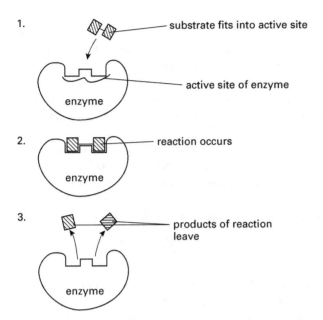

1. substrate fits into active site

active site of enzyme

enzyme

2. reaction occurs

enzyme

3. products of reaction leave

enzyme

Figure 3.1 How enzymes work.

Table 3.1 Comparison of the energy released by the oxidation of basic energy sources.

Source of energy	Amount of energy released
Carbohydrate	1g = 17kJ (4 kcal)
Protein	1g = 17kJ (4 kcal)
Fat	1g = 38kJ (9 kcal)

The main substance oxidised within the body is glucose, a sugar:

Glucose + Oxygen → Carbon dioxide + Water + *Energy* (2800kJ)

$C_6H_{12}O_6$ $6O_2$ $6CO_2$ $6H_2O$

The amount of energy produced is approximately 2800 kJ/mole of glucose. (A *mole* is a measure of the quantity of something, based on the number of molecules it contains.) In reality, this process is not simply one chemical reaction but a process of steps each speeded up or catalysed by a specific enzyme, and it takes place in all the cells of the body.

The glucose substrate may be obtained directly from digestion or it may be derived from its storage form, known as *glycogen*, which is stored in muscle and liver cells. Glycogen consists of long chains of glucose molecules joined together. Glycogen from the liver supplies glucose for all tissues in the body, including nerve and blood cells, whereas glycogen stored in muscles is used only for muscle contraction.

Adenosine triphosphate (ATP)

Energy is not a substance. It is released as a result of cellular respiration, in many stages, not all at one time. Some of this energy is released as heat, but most is stored as chemical energy in the form of *adenosine triphosphate (ATP)*, the energy currency of all cells. For example, when the horse moves its leg, energy is transferred from ATP to muscles to enable them to contract.

ATP is a molecule made within the mitochondria or 'power houses' of cells. It consists of an adenosine body with three phosphate groups attached. When one of the phosphates is detached, energy is released, leaving ADP (*adenosine diphosphate*) and a single phosphate. These single phosphates are later used to make more ATP.

ADENOSINE~P~P~P → ADENOSINE~P~P + P + Energy

Food contains substrates that can be used to release energy, with different foods containing different amounts of energy. For example, fat contains around twice as much energy as glucose. This has important implications when designing rations for horses requiring high levels of energy.

Anaerobic respiration and the oxygen debt

Respiration normally requires the presence of oxygen, and this is known as *aerobic* respiration. However, there are times when glucose may be broken down without the presence of oxygen, and this is known as *anaerobic* respiration. Anaerobic respiration produces less energy, but is very fast, so it is used only for short-term energy production – it may mean the difference between life and death for a zebra fleeing from a predator.

During strenuous exercise, horses cannot breathe in enough oxygen and the circulatory system is not able work fast enough to transport oxygen to the cells. A good example of a horse in this situation is the racehorse towards the end of a sprint (Figure 3.2). At some point the muscles start to produce energy by anaerobic respiration, without the presence of oxygen. This results in the muscles producing lactic acid as well, but not carbon dioxide.

Glucose → Lactic acid + *Energy* (210kJ)
$C_6H_{12}O_6$ $2C_3H_6O_3$

The amount of energy produced is approximately 210 kJ/mole of glucose, or less than one tenth of that produced by aerobic respiration.

During anaerobic respiration, lactic acid starts to accumulate in a horse's muscles, as shown above. Lactic acid may damage muscle cells,

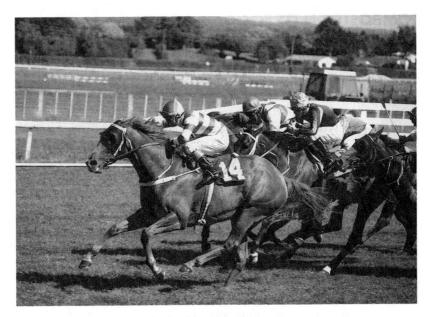

Figure 3.2   Racehorses at the finish line (sprinters).

making the muscles ache and feel heavy. When the race is over, this lactic acid has to be removed from the muscle cells before any long-lasting damage occurs. As the horse is 'blowing' following a race, more oxygen is taken in to break down the lactic acid to carbon dioxide and water. The amount of oxygen required to remove all the built up lactic acid is known as the *oxygen debt*. This debt has to be repaid immediately following a race.

For long-distance horses, lactic acid builds up more slowly, as the horse can breathe more efficiently over slower speeds. This results in less anaerobic respiration and in most cases the lactic acid may be broken down whilst the horse is still cantering – this is known as 'second wind'.

NUTRITION

In order to grow, horses must take substances into their bodies – a process known as *nutrition* or feeding. Horses, like most animals, feed on complex organic substances, breaking them down into soluble form in a process known as *digestion*. By contrast, plants make their own food by photosynthesis, taking in simple substances such as carbon dioxide and water and building them up to complex organic substances using energy from sunlight. The green pigment chlorophyll enables plants to use sunlight; hence most plants, including grass, are green in colour!

COMPOSITION OF FOOD

Horses need food for the following reasons:

- Provision of fuel for warmth and energy
- Provision of building blocks for growth
- Repair and replacement of worn out cells and tissues
- To help support a healthy immune system

The food the horse eats daily is known as the diet or ration. The diet should include the following important nutrients in the correct quantities:

- Water – provides fluid in which other molecules may move
- Carbohydrates – energy supply
- Fats – energy supply and help to waterproof the skin
- Proteins – building and repair of body tissues and enzymes
- Vitamins and minerals – for many different life functions

A diet that contains all these nutrients in the required proportions is known as a balanced diet. Minerals and vitamins are only required in relatively small amounts.

Water

Water is essential for life and must be included in the horse's diet. Approximately 70% of the body weight of the horse is made up of water. Horses take in water mainly by drinking, but some foods, such as fresh spring grass, contain more water than others. Horses consuming plenty of spring grass containing approximately 80–90% water will drink less water than those on a ration consisting mainly of dry hay at 10–15% water. Water is required for all life functions, and so they must have a clean supply of fresh water at all times, except after hard exercise, when it should be offered in frequent small amounts to prevent colic. Among its more important functions are:

- Temperature regulation
- Medium in which chemical reactions can take place
- Solvent in which substances may be dissolved and transported
- Gives cells their shape
- Excretion of toxins in the form of urine
- Lactation (the production of milk)

Carbohydrates

All carbohydrates contain carbon, hydrogen and oxygen. Perhaps the most well known carbohydrate is glucose ($C_6H_{12}O_6$). This formula shows that one glucose molecule contains:

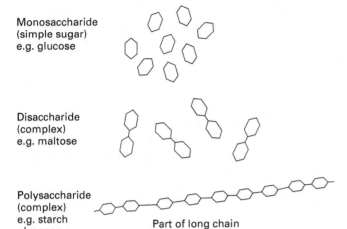

Monosaccharide
(simple sugar)
e.g. glucose

Disaccharide
(complex)
e.g. maltose

Polysaccharide
(complex)
e.g. starch
glycogen

Part of long chain

Figure 3.3 Simple and complex carbohydrates.

- 6 carbon atoms
- 12 hydrogen atoms
- 6 oxygen atoms

Carbohydrates fall into one of three groups (Figure 3.3):

- *Monosaccharides* – usually have a ring-shaped structure; form the building blocks of the more complex carbohydrates, e.g. glucose, fructose
- *Disaccharides* – formed from two monosaccharide units chemically bonded together, e.g. sucrose, maltose, lactose
- *Polysaccharides* – long chains of saccharide units, e.g. starch, glycogen

These three types of carbohydrate are interchangeable in that monosaccharides may be built up into disaccharides and polysaccharides while polysaccharides may be broken down into disaccharides and monosaccharides. Sugars are also known as *soluble* carbohydrates and polysaccharides as *insoluble* carbohydrates.

Monosaccharides

Monosaccharides are the simplest carbohydrates, or the simple sugars, such as glucose and fructose. These are single-unit sugars whose name derives from the Greek *mono* (single) and *sacchar* (sugar). Glucose is the main fuel for all cells, and has the chemical formula $C_6H_{12}O_6$. Fructose has the same formula, but the molecule is arranged slightly differently.

Disaccharides

Disaccharides consist of two monosaccharides, such as glucose, joined together. Maltose is a disaccharide made from two glucose molecules.

Sucrose ($C_{12}H_{22}O_{11}$), another common sugar, is a disaccharide obtained from one glucose molecule joined to one fructose molecule. Sucrose is the main carbohydrate found in plant sap, sugar beet and sugar cane. Lactose, or milk sugar, is another disaccharide.

Polysaccharides

Polysaccharides are long chains of sugar molecules, which may consist of a few hundred to several thousand units. *Starch* is a polysaccharide made from long chains of glucose molecules. Starch is the storage form of sugar in plants and is found in plant cells as starch grains. It is a concentrated form of energy. Cereals are a major source of starch.

Glycogen is another polysaccharide, again made up of long chains of glucose molecules, but containing more branches to the chain. Both starch and glycogen may be broken down into their constituent glucose units by breakage of the links joining them together. Horses have enzymes to break down these links.

Some polysaccharides are structural, in that they provide strength. An example of this is cellulose, which forms the fundamental structure of all plant-cell walls. Cellulose is also made up of many glucose units, but these are linked together differently from glycogen. The glucose links in cellulose cannot be broken down by the horse's own enzymes. The horse, like all herbivores needs micro-organisms, which produce the enzyme *cellulase*, to help them to break down cellulose. In horses these microbes live in the caecum and colon where they break down cellulose to the *volatile fatty acids* that are the end products – *acetic*, *propionic* and *butyric* acid. These are absorbed and used as energy sources by horses.

Fats

Fats and oils are essential to the horse and similar to carbohydrates, in that they are made up of carbon, hydrogen and oxygen. Fats are a concentrated source of energy. Much fat is stored under the skin to help keep the body warm.

Plant fats, for example those derived from sunflower, soya and corn, are normally liquid at room temperature and are known as oils. Fats and oils both have the same basic structure, but different physical characteristics.

Fats are made up of one *glycerol* molecule joined to one, two or three fatty acids, of which there are many. One of the most important of these is linoleic acid. This is an *essential* fatty acid in that the horse cannot manufacture it so it must be supplied in the horse's diet.

Fats are important in the diet for a number of reasons:

- As sources of essential fatty acids, e.g. linoleic acid
- As a concentrated source of energy (fat store)
- As a carrier for fat-soluble vitamins

Protein

The main structures of the horse's body, such as muscle, skin and connective tissue, are made up of protein. Protein is required for growth and repair of tissues, and to make enzymes. Proteins may also be used as an energy source, but only as a last resort, during times of starvation, for example.

Proteins are made of building blocks called *amino acids*. Horses can make some of these themselves, and so they are not required in the diet. They are therefore termed *non-essential* amino acids. Others cannot be made by the horse and must be supplied in the diet and are known as *essential* amino acids. Growing foals must be supplied with good-quality protein containing high levels of essential amino acids (Figure 3.4).

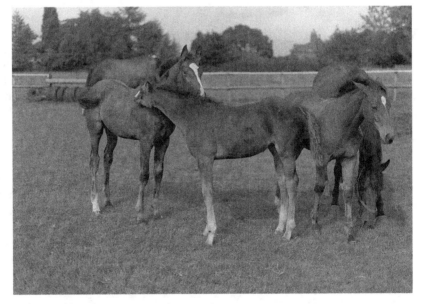

Figure 3.4 Growing foals must be supplied with good-quality protein to support their growth.

Minerals

Minerals, or mineral salts, contain chemical elements such as calcium and magnesium. These elements are required for many different functions within the body. Some are required only in tiny quantities and are known as *trace* elements.

Major minerals:

- Calcium
- Phosphorus
- Magnesium
- Sodium
- Potassium
- Chloride
- Sulphur

Trace minerals:

- Iron
- Copper
- Zinc
- Iodine
- Molybdenum
- Selenium
- Manganese
- Cobalt

Vitamins

Vitamins are organic nutrients that are required in metabolic reactions within the body, mostly helping enzymes. Although required in tiny amounts, they are vital for life. They can only function in solution: some dissolve in water (*water soluble*) and some in fat (*fat soluble*):

- Fat-soluble vitamins – A, D, E and K
- Water-soluble vitamins – C and B group

Fat-soluble vitamins are stored in the horse's body, mainly in the liver. Fresh green herbage is rich in this group of vitamins. Water-soluble vitamins cannot be stored in the body, and any excess will be excreted in the urine.

The functions, sources and deficiencies of vitamins and minerals are listed in Tables 3.2–3.5.

Table 3.2 Functions, sources and signs of fat-soluble vitamin deficiency.

Vitamin	Function	Sources	Signs of Deficiency
A (β-carotene)	Healthy eyes Immune system Growth and maintenance of body tissue	Grass Green forage	Lack of appetite Night blindness Poor growth Keratinisation of eyes Hoofs and skin in poor condition Infertility
D (sunshine vitamin)	Aids calcium and phosphorus absorption in the gut Bone formation Joint integrity	Synthesised in skin in the presence of sunlight Sun-dried hay	Bones fail to calcify, causing *rickets* in young horses and *osteomalacia* in older ones Swollen joints Fractures
E (tocopherol)	Muscle integrity Fat metabolism Acts with selenium as an antioxidant Reproduction	Alfalfa Green forage Cereals	Muscle disorders Infertility
K	Blood clotting	Produced by healthy hind-gut microbial population Leafy forage	True deficiency rare Levels can be assessed by measuring blood clotting time

ENERGY AND THE WORKING HORSE

Athletic horses have high energy requirements, mainly as fuel for the contraction and relaxation of muscles. The faster the speed the more energy required. The energy for this exercise is produced by the metabolism of glucose.

Respiration inside the muscle cells releases energy from glucose in the form of ATP. This ATP transfers energy directly to the muscle contraction system. The glucose is supplied by food. Excess food may be stored initially as fat and glycogen: the horse stores approximately 95% of body glycogen in muscle, and the remaining 5% in the liver; roughly 95% of body fat is stored in fatty (*adipose*) tissue and 5% in the liver.

Sources of energy for work

There are three main energy sources required for work, all of which supply energy for aerobic metabolism:

Table 3.3   Functions, sources and signs of deficiency of water-soluble vitamins.

Vitamin	Function	Sources	Signs of Deficiency
C (ascorbic acid)	Immune system Antioxidant Muscle and blood capillary integrity (Interacts with copper and iron)	Made in body tissues from glucose	Bleeding, ulcerated gums Internal bleeding
B$_1$ (thiamin)	Fat and carbohydrate, especially glucose, metabolism	Produced by healthy hind-gut microbial population	May be caused by eating bracken Loss of appetite Inco-ordination Staggering
B$_2$ (riboflavin)	Carbohydrate, protein and fat metabolism	Produced by healthy hind-gut microbial population	Poor growth rate Reduced utilisation of feed Possibly a factor in periodic ophthalmia
B$_6$ (pyridoxine – formerly vitamin H)	Carbohydrate, protein and fat metabolism Enzyme systems	Grass Green forage	Tryptophan and niacin cannot be utilised Poor growth Dermatitis Nerve degeneration
B$_{12}$ (cyanocobalamin)	Carbohydrate, protein and fat metabolism	Produced by healthy hind-gut microbial population, but requires cobalt for this	Poor growth Infertility Poor appetite Rough coat
Folic acid (folacin)	Maturation of red blood cells Interacts with vitamins B$_2$, B$_{12}$ and C	Grass Green forage Synthesised in hind-gut by healthy microbial population	Not described in horses
Biotin	Hoof-horn production Carbohydrate, protein and fat metabolism	Maize, yeast, soya Green forage	Poor hoof condition (crumbles at ground surface
Niacin (nicotinic acid)	Enzyme systems in all body cells Cell integrity and metabolism Carbohydrate, protein and fat digestion	Can be synthesised from the amino acid tryptophan Cereals	Not recorded in the horse
Pantothenic acid (calcium pantothenate)	Part of co-enzymes Carbohydrate, fat and protein digestion	Synthesised in hind-gut by healthy microbial population	No specific signs seen in horses

Table 3.4 Functions, sources and signs of deficiency of the major minerals.

Mineral	Function	Source	Signs of Deficiency
Calcium (Ca)	98% body Ca found in skeleton and teeth Blood clotting Nerve and muscle function Lactation	Alfalfa Limestone flour Green forage Sugar beet	Bone problems Rickets when young Osteomalacia when old Nutritional secondary hyperparathyroidism (big head disease) Enlarged joints Tying up
Phosphorus (P)	85% body P found in skeleton and teeth Energy production Enzyme systems	Cereals	Bone problems Rickets (young) Osteomalacia (old) Reduced or depraved appetite Poor growth
Magnesium (Mg)	60–70% body Mg found in skeleton and teeth Enzyme systems	Alfalfa Linseed	Weakness in limbs Muscle tremors Ataxia Sweating
Sodium (Na) **Chloride** (Cl) **Potassium** (K)	Body fluid regulation Muscle and nerve function Acid–base balance	Grass Hay Salt lick (NaCl only) Horses have a specific appetite for salt	Sweating Dehydration Muscle weakness Fatigue Exhaustion Depraved appetite
Sulphur (S)	Amino-acid synthesis Hoof and horn growth Enzyme systems Present in insulin	Grass	Poor hair and skin growth, including hooves

- Glycogen stores in the muscle
- Glucose from the blood
- Fatty acids from the blood

A further energy source, used by horses working at high speed, is anaerobic energy production from glucose or glycogen, which results in an accumulation of lactic acid (see Anaerobic respiration and the oxygen debt, pp. 30–31).

Glycogen is the storage form of glucose and is formed by the process of *condensation*. Glycogen is therefore stored with water – 1 g of glycogen stores 2.7 g of water:

Condensation

GLUCOSE $\rightleftarrows$ GLYCOGEN + WATER

Hydrolysis

Table 3.5 Function, sources and signs of deficiency of trace minerals.

Mineral	Function	Source	Signs of Deficiency
Iron (Fe)	60% of body Fe is used in haemoglobin synthesis Enzyme activation	Most natural feeds	Anaemia Weakness Pale mucous membranes Fatigue Poor growth Mares milk is low in Fe
Copper (Cu)	Haemoglobin synthesis Hair pigmentation Cartilage and elastin production Bone development Interacts with S and Mo Cell metabolism	Depends upon Cu content of soil in which feed is grown High Mo reduces Cu availability Yeast	Developmental orthopaedic disease Intermittent diarrhoea Loss of hair pigment Poor performance Poor growth Hair loss
Zinc (Zn)	Enzyme activator High Zn interferes with Cu utilisation Immune system	Cereals	Skin lesions Reduced appetite Poor growth
Iodine (I)	Required for synthesis of thyroid hormone (thyroxin) thus controlling metabolic rate	Most commercial feeds Seaweed products	Infertility Goitre
Molybdenum (Mo)	Enzyme activator	Often excessive in soil and therefore pasture Forage High Mo affects Cu availability	Deficiency symptoms not seen
Selenium (Se)	Antioxidant Interacts with vitamin E	Pasture Soil content varies Deficient areas are common USA has many areas where Se toxicity is common	Muscle disease Impaired cardiac function Respiratory problems Tying up
Manganese (Mn)	Carbohydrate, protein and fat metabolism Bone formation Lactation	Bran Grass (depending upon soil content)	Bone abnormalities Poor feed utilisation
Cobalt (Co)	Required for vitamin B_{12} synthesis	Trace levels present in most feeds	Anaemia Weight loss Poor growth

During exercise, glycogen stored in the muscle is used up first, and then circulating blood glucose is consumed. The resulting drop in blood glucose is detected by cells in the horse's pancreas that release the hormone *glucagon*, which circulates in the blood to the liver and stimulates it to convert its stored glycogen back into glucose. This is then released into the blood to travel to the muscles.

At the same time, during exercise, fat (*triglycerides*) that has been stored in the body in adipose tissue is broken down into fatty acids and glycerol. The fatty acids are transported to the muscles via the blood stream, where they are used by aerobic respiration to release energy. Fat releases just over twice as much energy as glucose; it does not require water for storage and therefore takes up less space. For endurance events, fatty acids will be the main source of energy. Fat is ideal for horses exercising at slow speeds over long distances.

As exercise continues, and stored sources of energy – glycogen and fatty acids – become depleted, the rate of glucose production slows, in part leading to fatigue.

ELECTROLYTES

When sodium chloride (NaCl – common salt) is dissolved in water, the two atoms separate. This process is known as ionisation and results in two charged particles or ions. Sodium has the positive charge Na^+ and chloride has the negative charge Cl^-. Sodium (Na), with the positive charge, is termed a *cation* because it will be attracted to a negative cathode whereas chloride (Cl), with the negative charge, is termed an *anion*, as it will be attracted to the positive anode.

Some ionic compounds, such as sodium chlorides, when in solution (dissolved) are known as electrolytes. This is because the solution can conduct electricity, giving these electrolytes important roles within the horse's body. These include:

- Conduction of electricity for the working nerve and muscle
- Exert osmotic pressure (see Chapter 1, pp. 13–14), keeping body fluids balanced
- May aid in acid–base balance

ACIDS AND ALKALIS

The number of hydrogen ions within a solution determines the acidity of that solution. Because the horse's biochemical reactions take place only within a narrow range of acidity, it is *vital* that the acidity level, or

Table 3.6   Normal pH values of different body fluids.

Body fluid	pH
Blood	7.35–7.45
Urine	4.5–8.0
Saliva	5.4–7.5
Gastric juice	1.5–3.5
Bile	6.0–8.5

normal concentration of hydrogen ions within the horse's body, is kept constant. The mechanisms that maintain this level are termed *homeostatic*, that is they regulate the horse's internal environment.

The scale by which levels of acidity in a solution are measured is called the *pH scale*:

- pH 7 is neutral
- pH 7–14 is alkali
- pH 0–7 is acid

The normal pH of any part of the horse's body may depend upon its function: for example, the horse's stomach contents have a low pH (they are acidic). Blood has a normal pH of 7.35–7.45. Much outside of this range and the health of the horse will be affected.

Many reactions within cells produce acids and bases (alkalis), and these have to be neutralised to maintain the correct pH for health. A delicate balance between acids and bases produced by the cells maintains the optimum pH. A base is a substance that will bind hydrogen ions and when dissolved in water produces an alkaline solution. When dissolved, some have the property of maintaining a constant pH. These are known as buffers. Buffers include some proteins, bicarbonates and phosphates. Buffers are vital for maintaining the correct pH. Examples of the normal pH of some of the horse's body fluids are shown in Table 3.6.

Alkalosis and acidosis

When the blood pH falls below 7.35 a complex buffer system within the blood, known as the *alkali reserve*, mops up the excess hydrogen ions. If the alkali reserve is used up, and there is an excess of free hydrogen ions within the blood, the horse is said to be in *acidosis*. If the reverse occurs, and the pH is higher than 7.45 and the increased alkali has mopped up all the *acid reserve*, the horse is said to be in *alkalosis*.

The horse's excretory system also helps to maintain blood pH within normal levels. The kidneys and the lungs, along with the buffer system, both help to maintain the correct acid–base balance.

Summary points

- Hundreds of thousands of chemical reactions occur simultaneously within the horse's cells
- Enzymes are biological catalysts that speed up the rate of chemical reactions
- All enzymes are proteins
- Respiration occurs at the cellular level and is the oxidation of food to provide energy
- ATP is the energy currency of all cells
- Three main energy sources for work include glycogen, glucose and fatty acids

The Digestive System

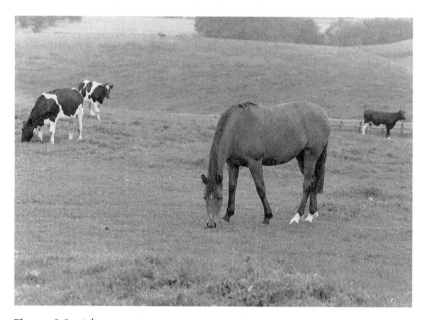

Figure 4.1 A horse grazing.

The digestive system is the collective name used to describe the alimentary canal and accessory organs associated with it such as the liver and the pancreas. The alimentary tract is the long tube through which food passes. It begins at the mouth, passes through the thorax, abdomen and pelvis and ends at the anus.

Horses consume huge quantities of grass (Figure 4.1), which contains a high proportion of cellulose, the structural carbohydrate found in plant cell walls. In common with other herbivores, horses do not produce the enzyme *cellulase*, which is required to break down this cellulose. Instead, they have developed a huge store of bacteria and other micro-organisms in the hind-gut (large intestine and caecum) that are able to produce this important enzyme.

The hind-gut micro-organisms break down cellulose by a process known as *fermentation* to energy-producing substances known as *volatile fatty acids*. The bacteria use some of the substances they produce for their own growth and they also use other nutrients such as proteins. Some of the products of bacterial fermentation are then absorbed by the caecum. Following break down of the food and removal of the nutrients from the gut, the remainder is excreted as waste.

The digestive system of the horse is unique and can be split into two parts (Figures 4.2 and 4.3):

- Foregut
- Hind-gut

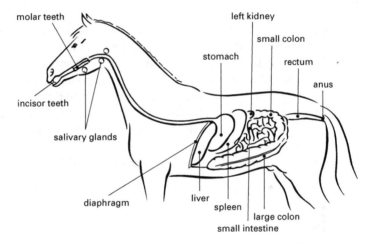

Figure 4.2 The horse's digestive system as viewed from the left side, showing the position of the gut within the abdomen.

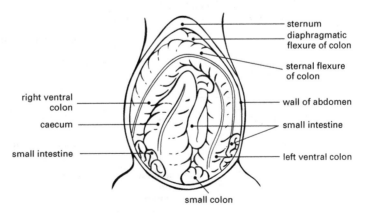

Figure 4.3 The horse's digestive system as viewed from beneath.

FOREGUT

The foregut is very similar to that of humans and pigs, while the hind-gut is similar to the rumen of a cow or a sheep. Figure 4.4 shows the differences between the digestive tracts of horses and ruminants.

The foregut consists of the mouth, pharynx, oesophagus, stomach and small intestine. The hind-gut consists of the caecum, large colon, small colon, rectum and anus. The horse's digestive tract is approximately 30 m or 100 ft long. In order to fit this great length into the abdominal space available, it is looped and loosely held in place by sheets of connective tissue known as the *mesentery* (Figures 4.2 and 4.3).

Mouth

Horses have strong, sensitive and mobile lips, enabling them to sort through food and graze close to the ground. The *incisor* teeth break off the food and the lips pass it onto the tongue. From here material is ground down by the *molars* through a series of chewing movements (side to side and up and down). Horses chew many more times when eating forage such as hay compared with concentrate feed. Saliva is produced while the horse is chewing, and this acts as a lubricant prior to swallowing. Unlike human saliva, the horse's saliva has no digestive activity, but it does contain *bicarbonate* to help neutralise the acid in the horse's stomach.

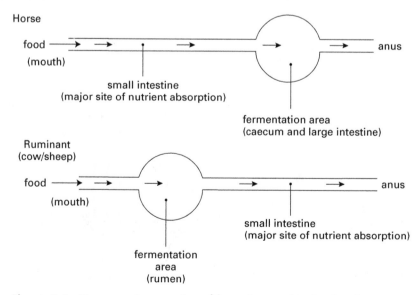

Figure 4.4   Diagrammatic comparison of the ruminant and equine digestive tracts.

The food is then swallowed: the highly-muscular tongue pushes the *bolus* (mouthful) of food to the back of the mouth, towards the pharynx; it passes into the pharynx and down the oesophagus. The epiglottis, a small flap of cartilage that forms part of the larynx, moves upwards and forwards to cover the *trachea* (windpipe) preventing food from entering the airways.

Oesophagus

The oesophagus is a muscular tube leading from the *pharynx* (mouth) to the stomach, the first main organ of digestion. Muscle fibres in the oesophagus contract and relax in turn creating a wave of movement, known as *peristalsis*, which pushes the food down the oesophagus (Figure 4.5). The lining of the oesophagus secretes mucus to aid the passage of the bolus of food to the stomach. Occasionally, food may become lodged or stuck in the oesophagus, and this is known as *choke*.

Stomach

Structure

The stomach is an elastic J-shaped organ (Figure 4.6). Food enters the stomach from the oesophagus through a valve known as the *cardiac sphincter*. The purpose of this valve is to prevent the stomach contents from moving back into the oesophagus, and it is so strong in the horse that the animal is unable to vomit. Food leaves the stomach through another valve, known as the *pyloric sphincter*, through which it enters the first part of the small intestine. The stomach wall consists of muscular layers with an inner mucous membrane lining.

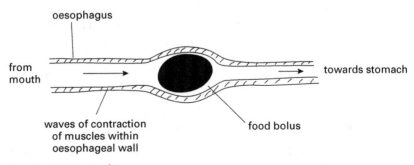

Figure 4.5 Peristalsis.

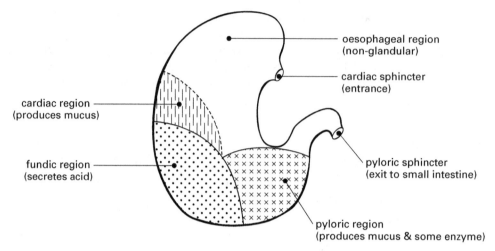

oesophageal region
(non-glandular)

cardiac sphincter
(entrance)

cardiac region
(produces mucus)

fundic region
(secretes acid)

pyloric sphincter
(exit to small intestine)

pyloric region
(produces mucus & some enzyme)

Figure 4.6 Regions of the horse's stomach.

Function

The functions of the stomach include:

- Begins protein digestion through the action of enzymes and hydrochloric acid
- Mixes food with gastric juices
- Lubricates food by secreting mucus
- Kills bacteria by secreting hydrochloric acid

The stomach of a 16 hh horse is about the size of a rugby ball and can stretch to hold about 8.5 litres. By contrast, the stomach of the cow may hold ten times as much. Because of this relatively small stomach volume, the horse has evolved as a trickle feeder, eating small amounts often, and using the stomach as a temporary holding vessel only.

Food begins the process of digestive break-down in the stomach due to enzymic and some microbial action. Gastric juice is produced continuously by the stomach in horses. Some 10–30 l of gastric juice is secreted daily and contains:

- *Hydrochloric acid* – neutralises bacteria and activates pepsin
- *Pepsin* – an enzyme that acts on protein to produce peptones, beginning digestion
- *Rennin* (foals only) – an enzyme that curdles milk, beginning its digestion

Small intestine

The length of the small intestine in the horse is approximately 20–27 m (65–88 ft) and has a capacity of 55–70 l. It runs from the stomach to the caecum and is split into three sections:

- *Duodenum*
- *Jejunum*
- *Ileum*

Structure

The duodenum is approximately 1 m long and forms an S-shaped bend in which sits the pancreas. The pancreatic and bile ducts enter the duodenum roughly 150 cm from the stomach. The jejunum is 20 m (65 ft) long and the ileum is 1–1.5 m or 3–5 ft long.

The walls of the intestine have four layers, including an outer muscular layer, a layer containing blood vessels, lymph vessels and nerves and an inner mucous membrane. The inner wall of the small intestine is covered with tiny finger-like projections known as *villi*. These increase the surface area for improved absorption and contain a network of blood capillaries and lymph vessels.

Function

The main function of the small intestine is to complete digestion of simple carbohydrates, fats and proteins. The end products are then absorbed through the villi into the blood capillaries. Digestion (Figure 4.7) and absorption (Figure 4.8) take place in the small intestine as peristaltic movements mix the food with intestinal and pancreatic juices as well as bile (see p. 50). Table 4.1 shows the digestive processes occurring in the different parts of the small intestine.

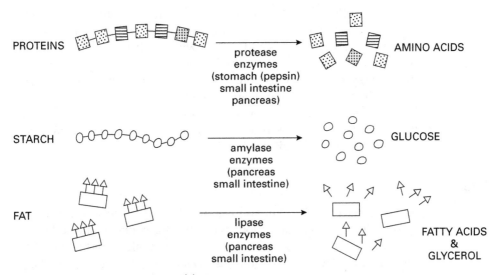

Figure 4.7 Digestive enzymes and their actions.

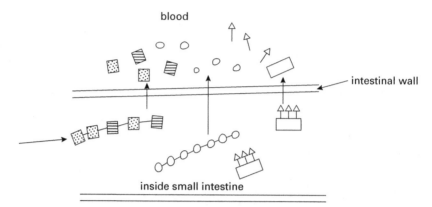

Figure 4.8 Movement of molecules from the small intestine to the blood.

Table 4.1 Digestion in the small intestine.

Organ	Secretion	Action
Duodenum	Pancreatic juice	
	Trypsin	Peptones → polypeptides
	Lipase	Fats → fatty acids & glycerol
	Amylase	Polysaccharides → disaccharides
	Bile	Emulsifies fats
Small intestine (villi)	Intestinal juice	
	Maltase	Disaccharides →
	Sucrase	monosaccharides
	Lactase	

The rate of passage of food through the small intestine is relatively fast, and food will reach the caecum in just over one hour. Non-fibrous soluble foods, e.g. starches and sugars, will be substantially digested in this relatively short time. The small intestine also helps to protect the digestive system from infection. It is the only part of the digestive tract with a direct link to the lymphatic system.

Enzymes of the small intestine require an alkaline environment to work effectively. This is produced by the effects of pancreatic juice from the pancreas and bile from the liver.

Bile

Bile is secreted by the liver and is a product of the break down of red blood cells. It is greenish yellow in colour. Bile contains salts, bile pigments (*bilirubin* and *biliverdin*), acids and water. Bile helps to neutralise the acid from the stomach and also *emulsifies* fat droplets, breaking larger ones into smaller droplets so that they can be more easily acted upon by enzymes. Unlike humans, the horse does not have a gall bladder in which to store bile; instead, bile trickles continuously into the duodenum from the bile duct.

HIND-GUT

The hind-gut is made up of the caecum, large colon, small colon and rectum. It is approximately 8 m (25 ft) long. Although the foregut of the horse is similar to that of other simple-stomached animals, the hind-gut is remarkably different.

It is in the hind-gut that the complex insoluble carbohydrates, cellulose and hemicellulose are digested by fermentation by micro-organisms. More than half the dry weight of the horse's droppings is bacteria. The number of micro-organisms in the digestive tract of the horse is enormous, numbering more than ten times the number of cells in the horse's body.

Caecum

The caecum is a large, blind-ended, comma-shaped sac at the end of the small intestine whose capacity is approximately 25–35 l. The caecum acts as a large fermentation vat, where fibrous parts of the food are mixed with digestive micro-organisms.

Large colon

The large colon holds approximately 100 l and is 3–4 m (10–13 ft) long. Its main function, and that of the caecum, is to house the billions of micro-organisms that digest cellulose and hemicellulose, producing volatile fatty acids. These micro-organisms are highly susceptible to dietary changes, and disruption of their balance can often result in digestive upsets such as diarrhoea or colic (Figure 4.9).

The other functions of the hind-gut are:

- Resorption of water
- Absorption of vitamins and salt
- Ridding the system of waste indigestible material

ACCESSORY ORGANS

There are two accessory organs which carry out functions associated with the digestive system of the horse. These are:

- Pancreas
- Liver

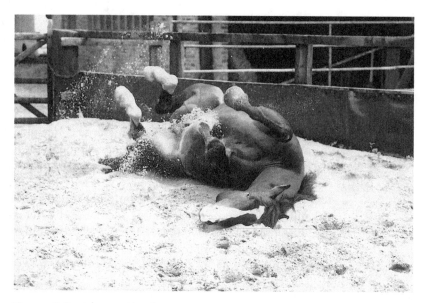

Figure 4.9 A horse with colic.

Pancreas

The pancreas is a gland situated behind the stomach between the spleen and duodenum. It secretes pancreatic juices into the duodenum through a tube known as the *pancreatic duct*.

The cells of the pancreas are divided into the *insulin-* and *glucagon-*producing cells of the islets of Langerhans, and a network of small alveoli, lined with cells producing digestive enzymes. Insulin and glucagon regulate blood sugar level following feeding, to maintain a normal range of blood glucose. The pancreas thus works with both the digestive system and the *endocrine* (hormone) system.

Liver

Structure

The liver is the largest gland in the horse's body (Figure 4.10). It is situated immediately behind the diaphragm and in front of the stomach and weighs 5–9 kg (12–20 lb).

The liver is supplied with blood from two sources: about 75% of it comes via the *hepatic portal vein* which arrives from the stomach and small intestine. This blood contains the products of digestion; the second, smaller, blood supply to the liver is from the *hepatic artery*, delivering oxygenated blood from the aorta.

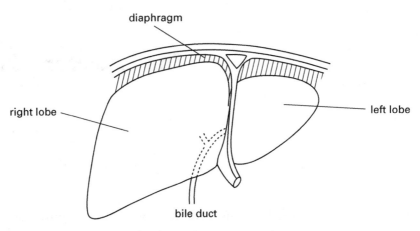

Figure 4.10 Structure of the horse's liver.

Liver tissue is made up of much smaller units known as liver lobules. These liver lobules are the sites of activity for the many functions of the liver. The liver is vital for cleansing and storage of substances in addition to production of bile and other essential substances.

Functions

- Removes toxins from harmful substances such as drugs
- Removes nitrogen from amino acids
- Stores glycogen, vitamins A, D, E and K, iron and fats
- Produces heat, vitamins A and D, heparin, plasma proteins (albumin and globulin), prothrombin and fibrinogen, bile, uric acid and urea
- Converts glycogen to glucose, glucose to glycogen, stored fats into other fats such as cholesterol
- Metabolises protein – builds up and breaks down protein

Summary points

- The horse is a hind-gut fermenter, eating forage little and often
- The digestive system converts food and water to nutrients and waste
- Enzymes are used to break down foods into smaller units that are then absorbed
- Accessory organs are the pancreas and liver
- Horses have a relatively small stomach
- Horses do not have a gall bladder as they are trickle feeders
- The caecum is the main site for microbial digestion of cellulose

---

The Excretory System

5

The horse's body must continually rid itself of unwanted and sometimes toxic waste substances, otherwise the working environment of its cells would soon become unsustainable. The process by which any organism does this is known as *excretion*.

All living cells produce waste substances during metabolism. For example, a waste product such as carbon dioxide produced from respiration within a cell is an excretory product. However, waste such as that found in the horse's droppings is simply indigestible material and bacteria, none of which have been in involved in metabolic reactions within cells – the material has passed unchanged through the horse's digestive system. This type of waste removal is known as *evacuation* or *egestion* and should not be confused with excretion.

EXCRETORY PRODUCTS

The horse's excretory products are shown in Table 5.1.

- *Carbon dioxide* – This is produced during cellular respiration and is excreted, via the lungs, when the horse breathes out.
- *Nitrogenous waste* – Horses need protein in their diet, but if they eat more than they need the extra cannot be stored within the body and has to be removed. This excess protein is broken down in the liver, by a process known as *deamination*, to carbohydrate (or fat) and urea

Table 5.1 The horse's excretory products.

Excretory product	Where made	Process	How excreted
Carbon dioxide	All living cells	Respiration	From lungs
Nitrogenous waste	Liver	Deamination	From kidneys (urine)
Bile pigments	Liver and spleen	From haemoglobin	In bile (droppings)

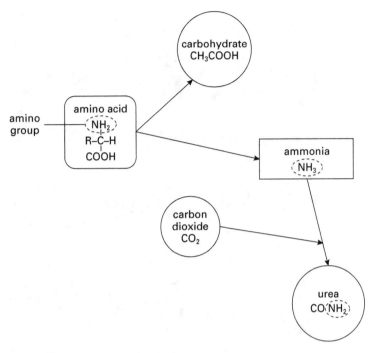

Figure 5.1   Break down of amino acids to urea.

(Figure 5.1). Urea contains the nitrogen part of protein and dissolves in the blood before being taken to the kidneys. A small amount of urea may also be excreted in the horse's sweat.

- *Bile pigments* – When red blood cells age and begin to deteriorate they must be broken down in the liver and spleen. The iron from the haemoglobin they contain is kept to be recycled. The rest of the haemoglobin is turned into bile pigments and excreted via the digestive tract in bile. Bile is secreted into the duodenum of the digestive tract and helps to break down fat before being excreted in the faeces.
- Other substances exist in delicate balances within the horse's body and these include salt and water.

WATER

Horses generally take in more water then they need, particularly when grazing lush spring pasture, which contains a large amount of water. Surplus water within the body will need to be removed in order to maintain the blood concentration at the right level. The process by which horses gain and lose water in order to maintain the correct concentration of blood is known as *osmoregulation*. Horses gain water in the following ways:

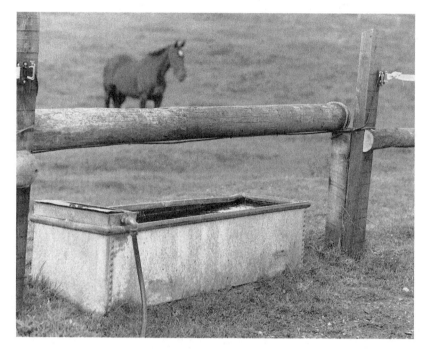

Figure 5.2 A water trough supplies horses with adequate drinking water.

- Drinking (Figure 5.2)
- Eating – grass, haylage, soaked beet pulp, etc.
- Respiration – water is produced as a by-product (see Chapter 3, pp. 28–31)

Horses lose water in the following ways:

- Urinating
- Sweating
- Breathing out (lungs)
- In droppings

Salt and water are both involved in osmoregulation and this process takes place in the urinary system (see below).

Controlling water balance

The control of body water balance is crucial for all animals.

If the horse's body is short of water the concentration of salts within the blood will be too high. This is detected by special brain cells, which send instructions to the *pituitary gland* (see Chapter 11, pp. 135–6) to secrete a hormone known as *antidiuretic hormone* (ADH) into the blood. ADH counteracts *diuresis* which is the increased outflow of urine from

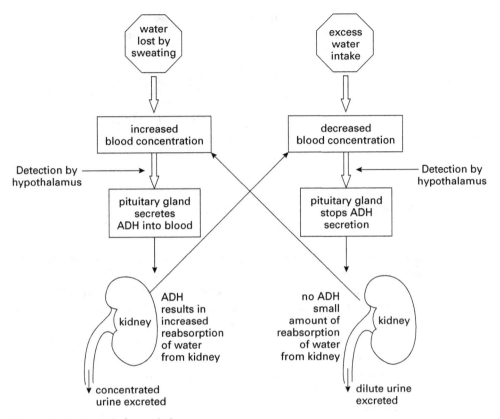

Figure 5.3   Control of water balance.

the body. It is carried to the kidneys, which respond to the hormone by reabsorbing water thus reducing water output in the urine. At the same time, the horse will feel thirsty so that it will drink, if water is available. The control of water balance in horses is shown in Figure 5.3.

When horses are deprived of water, the quantity of urine produced is low and the concentration of that urine is high. A mechanism known as the sodium pump, which is situated in a loop of the tubule known as the loop of Henlé, is responsible for the addition or removal of water and therefore the concentration of urine (see below).

URINARY SYSTEM – THE KIDNEYS

The horse has a pair of kidneys, which lie on either side of the horse's body, midway between the withers and the croup, underneath the spinal column. The left kidney lies slightly farther back towards the last rib, whereas the right kidney lies under the last three ribs. The kidneys

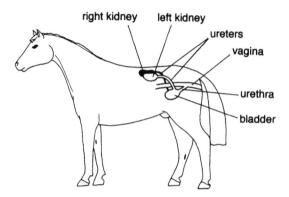

Figure 5.4   Position of the horse's urinary organs.

are extremely well protected in this position (Figure 5.4). The horse is unusual in that each kidney is shaped differently from the other – the left one is bean shaped and the right is heart shaped. There are often large collections of fat around them, which also affords them protection.

Kidneys are organs that filter plasma from the blood (see The nephron, below). They are highly efficient sieves, which allow the passage of smaller particles through but keep larger particles, such as blood cells, out. From the substances that are filtered through, the kidneys can selectively reabsorb water and other useful substances so that they are not wasted by being excreted in urine.

The structure of a kidney is shown in Figure 5.5. Every day, approximately 1000–2000 l of fluid are delivered to a horse's kidneys, of which only 5–15 l are excreted in the form of urine, the kidneys having reabsorbed most of the fluid. If the kidneys did not reabsorb this fluid, horses would lose their entire water and salt content in less than half a day.

Kidneys perform a number of functions in their homeostatic role:

- Maintain the volume of extracellular fluid
- Maintain the balance of ions in extracellular fluid
- Maintain pH and osmotic balance in extracellular fluid
- Excrete toxic substances, e.g. urea

The nephron

Structure

Apart from blood vessels and a small amount of connective tissue, the kidney consists of a mass of tubules known as *nephrons*. Each nephron is a tube which starts in the *cortex* of the kidney as a blind-ended thin-walled

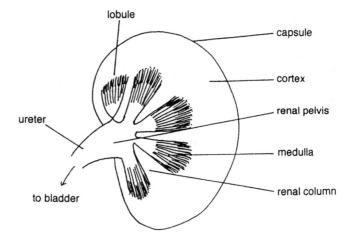

The lobular form of the kidney is partially obliterated in the horse

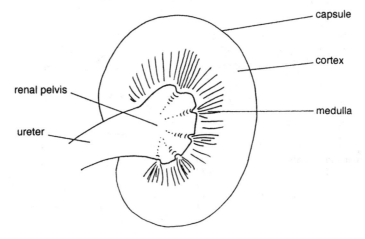

Figure 5.5   Structure of the kidney.

sac (Bowman's capsule) into which a knot of blood vessels passes (the *glomerulus*). Bowman's capsule and the glomerulus are known together as a Malphigian body. From the Malphigian body, the hollow tube of the nephron is known as a *renal tubule*. It is the tubule that coils and loops and passes between the cortex and *medulla* and back again. The horse's kidney has approximately 2.5 million nephrons (Figure 5.6).

Function

The main functions of the kidney tubules are to filter out unwanted waste products *from* the blood and to reabsorb large volumes of

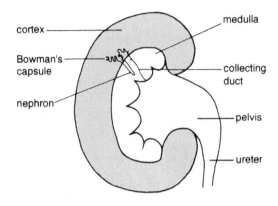

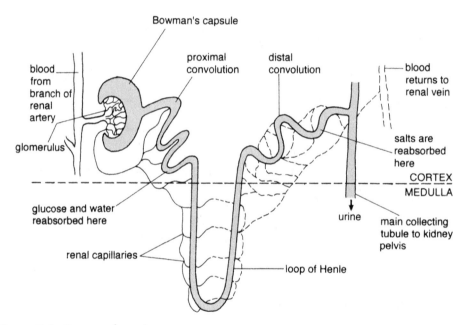

Figure 5.6 Structure of a nephron.

fluids and the majority of substances dissolved in that fluid *into* the blood.

Bowman's capsule is a highly-efficient filter. Blood passes into the glomerulus at high pressure from the renal artery, and substances that are not too large, such as dissolved salts, glucose, amino acids and urea, pass through the capsule into the tube or tubule. Substances, such as blood cells and protein molecules, which are too large, stay in the blood. If there is a fall in blood pressure, for example if the horse is haemorrhaging (bleeding), then the filtration process may stop and no urine will be formed.

As long as there is no damage to the tubule, or an abnormally high concentration of a substance in the blood, all the glucose and amino acids and a great proportion of the potassium and sodium, are filtered off in the glomerular filtrate and reabsorbed early on in the tubules of the kidney. This reabsorption is an active process, requiring energy, but it is accompanied by the passive reabsorption of water.

Sodium and potassium

In addition to regulating body water, the kidneys are responsible for regulating the concentration of body salts (*electrolytes*), such as sodium and potassium, in the blood. This regulation takes place in the tubule mechanism.

Aldosterone is a hormone secreted by the kidneys. This hormone regulates the movement of sodium from the nephron to the blood. If blood sodium levels fall, aldosterone is released into the blood resulting in more sodium passing from the nephron back to the blood. In addition, water flows back into the blood by osmosis.

The horse is also able to regulate its body salt levels by its behaviour. When sodium levels drop, the horse senses this and tries to make good the loss by actively seeking out and ingesting salt by licking soil and fences.

Acid–base balance

Chemical reactions are continually taking place in every cell of the body and, as a result of this metabolic activity, the cells are continuously producing acids. Acids may also derive from the horse's diet. However, in spite of all this acid production, the pH of the blood plasma and other body fluids must remain constant around neutral. The kidney has an important role to play in acid–base balance by controlling the excretion of bicarbonate in the urine, making it more or less acidic and compensating for alkalosis or acidosis in the horse's body (see Chapter 3, pp. 42–3).

Urination

This is the term used for the elimination of urine from the bladder.

The urine produced by the kidneys in the renal tubules is transferred to the *ureters* and carried by them to the bladder, which acts as a storage vessel for urine. It has elastic walls so that it can expand to hold more urine when necessary. Leading out of the bladder is a tube called the *urethra* with a tight sphincter muscle at the top. When the bladder is full this sphincter muscle opens to allow evacuation of urine.

Horses tend to urinate (stale) at rest when on grass or bedding, and tend to do so four to six times a day. They adopt a typical posture for this, with the hind legs spread apart and the horse leaning slightly forward. There is contraction of the muscles of the abdominal wall and the tail is raised. Often, horses will grunt and groan when urinating. This is normal and does not indicate discomfort or pain.

Summary points

- The kidneys filter the blood of potentially harmful substances
- The kidneys help control water balance and regulate important body salts
- The kidneys produce urine through a filtration process
- The horse excretes urine via the bladder

The Musculoskeletal System

THE SKELETON

The skeleton is a hardened framework of bone and cartilage that supports and protects muscles and vital organs of the horse's body. The skeleton functions to:

- Provide rigidity and shape to the body
- Protect vital organs
- Make red and white blood cells and platelets in the marrow
- Allow *locomotion* (movement of the whole horse)
- Provide a store of calcium and phosphorus
- Provide attachments for muscles allowing movement

The skeleton consists of bone, cartilage and joints and may be divided into two parts:

- *Axial* skeleton, which consists of those parts of the skeleton that lie along the main axis of the body – skull, vertebral column, ribs, sternum – the main functions of which are to support the body and protect organs
- *Appendicular* skeleton, consisting of those parts of the skeleton that attach to the axial skeleton – shoulder girdle, fore and hind limbs, pelvic girdle – the main function of which is to bring about movement and locomotion

The horse's skeleton is shown in Figure 6.1.

Bone

Most of the horse's skeleton is made of bone, which consists mainly of mineral salts, such as calcium phosphate and small amounts of magnesium, which give bone its hardness, and contains 25% water. But bone also contains collagen, which gives it a small amount of elasticity. If calcium is removed in the laboratory by treating the bone with acid, the bone becomes rubbery and floppy.

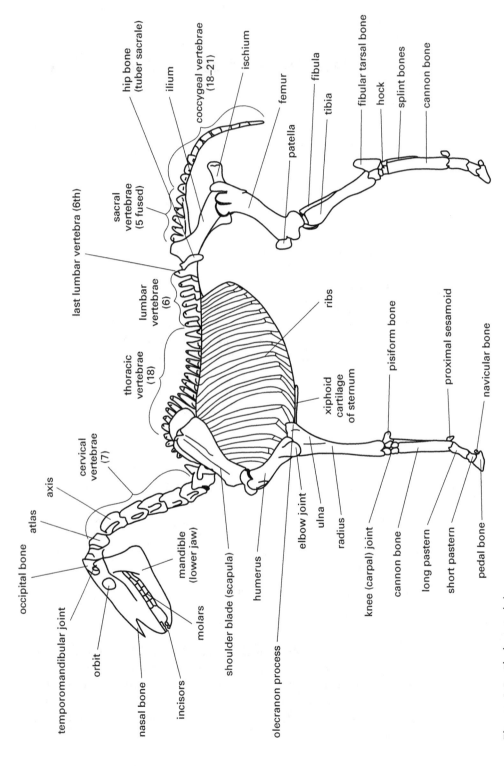

Figure 6.1   The horse's skeleton.

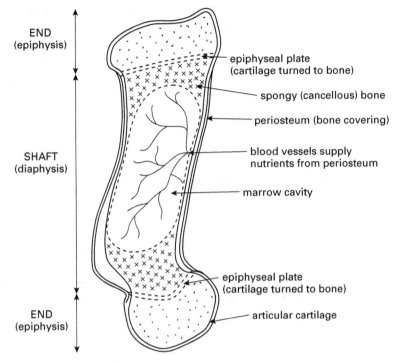

END
(epiphysis)

epiphyseal plate
(cartilage turned to bone)

spongy (cancellous) bone

periosteum (bone covering)

SHAFT
(diaphysis)

blood vessels supply
nutrients from periosteum

marrow cavity

epiphyseal plate
(cartilage turned to bone)

END
(epiphysis)

articular cartilage

Figure 6.2 A typical long bone.

Bone is a living tissue with living bone cells known as *osteoblasts* supplied with food and oxygen by blood vessels. It is the osteoblasts that produce calcium phosphate crystals and with collagen. Stress on a bone is detected by these bone cells which respond by making more bone tissue for added strength.

Bone tissue also varies considerably in density – the nearer to the surface of the bone the more compact it is. Many bones, including the ribs and long bones, have a central cavity which contains marrow, the source of red and white blood cells, platelets and also functions as a storage area for fats. The structure of a typical long bone is shown in Figure 6.2.

There are 206 bones in the horse's body, the smallest being the *stapes*, or stirrup bone, in the middle ear. There are five different types of bone, which are classified according to their shape:

- *Long bones* – the levers of the horse's body, which allow movement, particularly of the limbs; they include the radius, tibia, femur, humerus and cannon bones
- *Short bones* – strong and compact such as those found in the knee and hock
- *Flat bones* – protective bones with broad flat surfaces, such as the skull, scapula (shoulder), pelvis and sternum

- *Irregular bones* – do not fit into any of the above categories, for example the vertebrae, maxilla and mandible
- *Sesamoid bones* – bones within tendons or ligaments; provide strength to tendons where they change direction, for example in the fetlock joints

These bones may consist of two different types of bone tissue:

- Compact
- Cancellous

The amount of each type of tissue found within the bone depends upon the type and function of the bone concerned.

Compact bone

Compact bone has a honeycomb appearance when viewed under the microscope, even though it appears dense to the human eye. Compact bone is harder than cancellous bone and forms a supporting sheath to most bones, and is also found within the shaft of long bones. Compact bone contains Haversian canals, which run lengthways through the tissue, containing blood, lymph and nerves.

Cancellous bone

Also known as spongy bone because it has the appearance of a sponge, this bone has holes in it making it lighter. Cancellous bone is found at the ends of the long bones and also in flat, irregular and sesamoid bones.

Bone growth

As a foal grows in size, so must the skeleton grow to support its body. In the unborn foal, bone begins as cartilage. Specialised cells called osteoblasts, which lay down the matrix for bone, then invade this cartilage. Minerals are then deposited in the matrix, by a process known as calcification, resulting in strong bone.

Calcification is almost complete by the time the foal is born, however there are parts of the bone that allow it to continue to grow in length and width as the foal matures. The increase in length of bone takes place at two narrow bands of cartilage, at either end of the bone, known as the *epiphyseal growth plates* (Figure 6.3).

Cartilage grows continuously on the side of the growth plate closest to the end of the bone. At the same time the cartilage on the other side, i.e. nearest to the middle of the bone or shaft side, is converted to bone following the invasion of osteoblasts (Figure 6.3). Gradually the

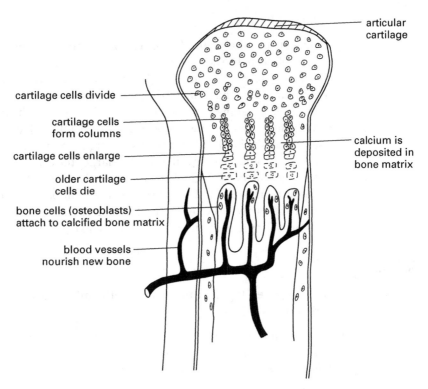

Figure 6.3 The area of bone growth in a long bone.

osteoblasts catch up with the cartilage so that the bone is the correct length. At this point the growth or epiphyseal plate is said to have 'closed'.

The different growth plates close at different times in horses:

- Just above knee (lower end of radius) – 2.5 years
- Lower end of cannon bone – 9–12 months
- Fetlock – 8–9 months

The growth plates of the distal radius, however, do not close until well into the racing career of a Thoroughbred flat-racing horse and this can create lumpy bony swellings above the knee when the horse is subjected to too much work, particularly on hard or firm ground.

Bone also increases in width or diameter. The bone coating, or *periosteum*, contains osteoblasts that lay down new layers of bone over old. At the same time, cells called *osteoclasts* break down bone and reabsorb it from the inside of the bone cavity so that the wall of the shaft does not become too thick and heavy.

Bone remodelling

Throughout the life of the horse its bone is remodelling, creating a balance between break down of old bone and production of new. Remodelling helps the horse's skeleton to adapt to stress and also acts as a mineral store, which can be dipped into at times of need.

Remodelling begins in the foal at around three months of age. The newly-formed bone begins to rearrange itself into Haversian canals. These are canals that run lengthways through compact bone and they contain nerves and blood capillaries. The larger the canal the less dense and compact the bone. If the Haversian canals are formed too quickly without adequate mineral content, the bone will become porous and not as strong as dense bone. The diet must have adequate calcium and phosphorus for proper bone remodelling to take place.

Joints

Bones are joined together in joints in different ways. There are three different types of joint:

- *Fixed*, or fibrous
- *Cartilaginous*, or slightly moveable
- *Synovial*, or freely moveable

Fixed, or fibrous, joints have no movement. They are made up of fibrous tissue which joins the ends of bones such as the plates in the skull or in the pelvic girdle.

Cartilaginous joints are slightly moveable. They move by compression of the cartilage and consist of a pad of fibrocartilage between bones. Pads such as these are found between the vertebrae of the spine.

The structure of a typical, synovial joint is shown in Figure 6.4. They are freely moveable and are modified to be shock absorbers and allow smooth movement. The synovial membrane that lines the joint makes synovial fluid, which is slightly viscous in nature, to help lubricate it.

There are four different types of synovial joint in horses:

- *Ball and socket* – the most moveable, e.g. shoulder and hip joints
- *Hinge* – allow movement in one plane only, giving flexion and extension, e.g. joints between the pedal bone, short pastern and long pastern bones
- *Gliding* – the least moveable; allow the bones to glide over each other, e.g. in the *carpal* (knee) and *tarsal* (hock) joints
- *Pivot* – allow movement round one axis and a rotational movement, e.g. the joint between the atlas and axis, the first two cervical vertebrae, which allows the horse's head to rotate to a limited extent (*atlantoaxial joint*)

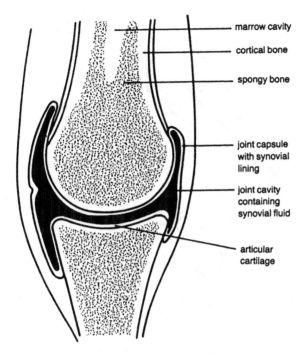

marrow cavity

cortical bone

spongy bone

joint capsule
with synovial
lining

joint cavity
containing
synovial fluid

articular
cartilage

Figure 6.4 Structure of a typical synovial joint.

The bones are held in position at joints by the fibrous *joint capsules* which cover the joints and by the ligaments and muscles which run from one bone to another (there are no muscles below the knee and hock). Some ligaments are located within the joint and others outside of it. The ligaments are responsible for limiting movement at the joint and maintaining the structure of the joint.

Vertebral column

The more common name for the vertebral column is the spine. This is the central part of the skeleton, which supports the horse's head and spinal cord. The vertebral column houses the vital nerves of the spinal cord, which carries impulses from the brain. In horses the vertebral column includes the vertebrae of the neck, withers, back and tail.

The vertebral column may be divided into five regions:

- Neck – 7 cervical vertebrae
- Upper back – 18 thoracic vertebrae
- Loins – 6 lumbar vertebrae
- Croup – 5 fused sacral vertebrae
- Tail – 15–20 coccygeal vertebrae

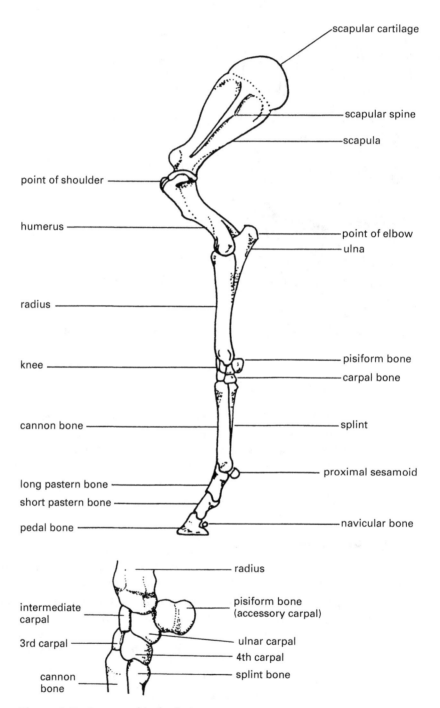

Figure 6.5 Structure of the forelimb.

The vertebrae make up a long chain, forming a 'tube' within it to house the spinal cord. At each vertebra a pair of spinal nerves exits from the spinal cord to supply every part of the horse's body. Muscles are attached by ligaments to the vertebrae, allowing the horse to move.

The horse has very limited movement of the spine from the withers to the loins.

Appendicular skeleton

The appendicular skeleton is attached to the axial skeleton by the *pelvic* and *pectoral girdles*. The horse does not have a collar bone, and therefore the pectoral girdle is attached to the spine, ribs and sternum by muscles and ligaments only. This means that the forehand of the horse is designed to support the body and absorb concussion and not to propel the horse forwards.

The lower limbs of the horse are adapted for speed in that they are long levers attached to muscles higher up in the limbs via long tendons. This gives a long stride enabling the horse to cover more ground with each step.

Forelimb

The forelimb consists of the following bones and joints (Figure 6.5):

- Scapula
- Shoulder
- Humerus
- Elbow
- Radius and ulna
- Knee (carpus)
- Cannon and two splint bones (metacarpals)
- Fetlock
- Long pastern, short pastern, pedal bone (three phalanges)
- Sesamoid bones (two sesamoids and the navicular bone)

The humerus is one of the strongest bones in the horse's body. Its angulations make it ideal for shock absorption. The horse's radius and ulna are fused together (unlike those of humans) to prevent any twisting of the forearm. The horse's knee is equivalent to the human wrist and consists of seven or eight small carpal bones. The knee's structure also allows it to function as a shock absorber. The cannon bone is weight-bearing and has the typical hard, supportive compact bone sheath surrounding a core of spongy cancellous bone.

The joint between the cannon bone and the long pastern bone is known as the *fetlock* joint. This is subjected to a large amount of mechanical stress and a great deal of movement.

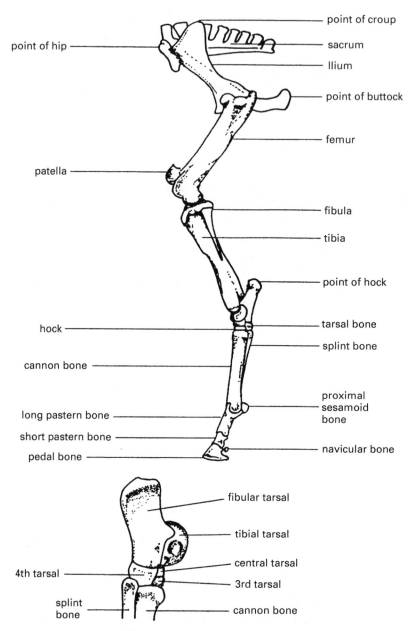

Figure 6.6   Structure of the hind limb.

Hind limb

The hind limb consists of the following bones and joints (Figure 6.6):

- Pelvis
- Hip
- Femur
- Stifle joint and patella
- Tibia and fibula
- Hock (tarsus)
- Cannon and two splint bones (metatarsals)
- Fetlock
- Long pastern, short pastern, pedal bone (three phalanges)
- Sesamoid bones (two sesamoids and the navicular bone)

The femur is the strong bone that runs between the hip and stifle joints and is adapted for attachment of the muscles of the hindquarter. The patella is called the kneecap in humans. It is associated with the stifle, which is the joint between the femur and the tibia. The tibia runs between the stifle and hock joints, but the fibula, which in some species is an individual bone, is small and almost vestigial in the horse.

The horse's hock, or tarsus, consists of six or seven short flat bones arranged in three rows. A long bony process gives rise to the point of hock. Below the hock the arrangement of bones is the same as the forelimb.

Tendons and ligaments

Tendons

Tendons are fibrous cords of connective tissue that attach skeletal muscles to bones (unlike ligaments, which connect bone to bone). Some tendons, particularly those in the lower limbs, are enclosed in self-lubricating sheaths that protect against friction. Tendons are strongly linked to bones by perforating fibres or Sharpey's fibres. These are extensions of the collagen fibres that mostly make up the tendon, and they pass through the bone's outer layer, or periosteum, and are then embedded in the outer bone itself. This gives a strong anchorage, keeping the tendons firmly attached during movement.

Tendons are relatively inelastic but they are made up of crimped fibres giving a slight ability to lengthen. Providing the tendon is not overloaded it returns to the crimp formation after the load is removed.

Ligaments

Ligaments originate from bone and attach to bone, i.e. they attach bone to bone. Ligaments are even less elastic than tendons and have no muscular attachments. Overstretching of a limb joint is particularly common in horses and this can result in damage to the inelastic supporting ligaments, causing a sprain.

The *suspensory ligament* of the horse differs from other ligaments in that it is a modified muscle. It contains some muscular tissue, giving considerable elasticity compared to other ligaments. The suspensory ligament lies between the deep digital flexor tendon and the cannon bone, and is often mistaken for the splint bone, as it feels rigid when the horse bears weight on that leg. At the levels of the sesamoid bones it splits into two branches, passing forwards to join the extensor tendon at the front of the pastern. The suspensory ligament is part of the *stay apparatus* and its function is to suspend and prevent over extension of the fetlock joint.

The hoof

The bones of the horse's hoof are equivalent to the bones of the middle finger of humans. These bones have various names:

- First, second and third phalanges
- Proximal, middle and distal phalanges
- Long pastern, short pastern and pedal bone (most commonly used)

There are joints between these bones: the joint between the cannon bone and the long pastern bone is known as the *fetlock* joint; the joint

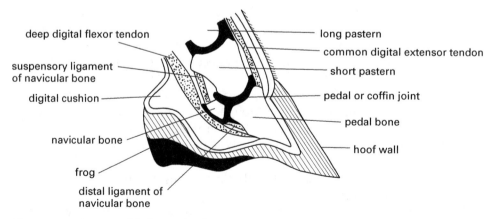

deep digital flexor tendon

suspensory ligament of navicular bone

digital cushion

navicular bone

frog

distal ligament of navicular bone

long pastern

common digital extensor tendon

short pastern

pedal or coffin joint

pedal bone

hoof wall

Figure 6.7 Structure of the horse's hoof.

between the long and short pastern is known as the *pastern* joint; the joint between the short pastern and the pedal bone is called the *coffin* joint. The hoof capsule itself surrounds the pedal bone and part of the short pastern bone (Figure 6.7).

The horse's hoof is a highly-specialised structure whose function is to support the horse's weight, absorb concussion and resist wear. It is a continuation of modified skin, similar to horns and claws in other animals.

The external hoof is continuous with the epidermis and the internal hoof, or *corium*, is modified from the deeper layer of skin. The corium is the sensitive part of the hoof.

The hoof wall grows from the coronary band down the front of the pedal bone. It consists of approximately 25% water and is thicker at the toe than the heel. The toe is also harder than the heel allowing the heel to expand. It takes approximately six months for the heel to grow from top to ground level, and 9–12 months for the toe.

The horn, which makes up the external hoof, consists of epithelial cells in the form of horny tubules, which are impregnated with the protein *keratin*. The wall is covered by a thin layer of epidermis known as the *periople*. This is carried down the front of the hoof wall as the hoof grows and helps to balance moisture in and out of the hoof. The external hoof does not have a blood supply and is insensitive to pain, which is why the horse does not wince when shoes are nailed on correctly.

The external underside of the hoof is shown in Figure 6.8, showing sites of common problems. The wall at the heel is turned forwards to form bars. These bars give strength to the heel and allow the hoof to withstand the weight of the horse. The bars also allow for expansion

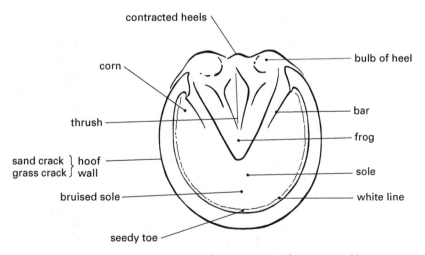

Figure 6.8 Underside of the horse's hoof, showing sites of common problems.

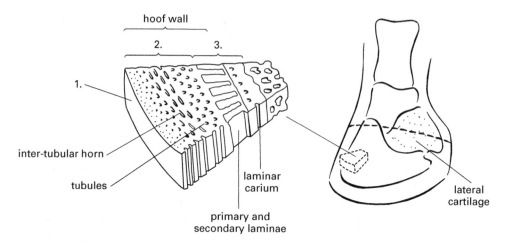

1. Stratum externum (periople and tectorial layer)
2. Stratum medium (tubular layer)
3. Stratum internum (laminar layer containing interlocking laminae)

Figure 6.9   The interlocking laminae.

when the horse's weight lands on the hoof. The bars should be allowed to grow to prevent the heels contracting.

The internal surface of the hoof wall is covered with 500–600 horny *laminae*, or leaves, each of which has 100–200 secondary laminae. These horny laminae provide a very strong bond by interweaving with the sensitive laminae attached to the pedal bone (Figure 6.9). The white line on the underside of the hoof shows the junction between the insensitive and the sensitive laminae.

Weight bearing

When the horse puts weight on the hoof, it presses down on the pedal bone. The pedal bone, in its turn, presses on arteries and veins forcing blood back up the leg – this effect is known as the *foot pump*. There is a hydraulic effect due to some resistance within the blood vessels which helps to absorb concussion. Some concussion is also absorbed by the hoof wall which bows as it receives the weight and the heels spread.

The *frog* is a wedge of soft elastic horn containing approximately 45% moisture and situated between the bars. It has a central groove and its main functions are to absorb concussion, assist circulation and aid grip. As the frog hits the ground it is squeezed and expands, placing pressure on the *digital cushion*. The digital cushion is a wedge-shaped fibroelastic pad situated in the back part of the hoof above the front and below the deep digital flexor tendon. This in turn squeezes the *lateral cartilages,* which lie on either side of the digital cushion, and the wall of the hoof expands.

Summary points on the skeleton

- The skeleton supports and protects vital body organs
- The skeleton is divided into two parts, the axial and appendicular skeletons
- Joints are where two bones meet
- Synovial joints are shock absorbers
- The vertebral column, or spine, houses the spinal cord
- The external hoof is continuous with the horse's skin
- The hoof is designed to absorb concussion
- Tendons join muscle to bone
- Ligaments join bone to bone
- The suspensory ligament is a modified muscle

THE MUSCLES

Muscles enable horses to move – to search for food and to escape from danger to give two simple examples. Muscles enable horses, with training, to carry out highly intricate manoeuvres such as those carried out by advanced dressage horses (Figure 6.10).

The muscle system comprises the muscles of the horse's body and their attachments, tendons and fascia. The function of muscle is to contract and by doing so initiate movement. It contracts following nervous stimulation from the brain. This causes the muscle to become shorter and fatter, and as it contracts it exerts a pull on its attachments to other parts of the horse's musculoskeletal system. Muscles also help to stabilise joints, maintain posture and, through shivering, aid in temperature control.

The smallest muscle in the horse's body is skeletal and attached to the stapes in the horse's ear. The largest and longest muscle in the horse's body is the *longissimus dorsi.*

A muscle is a group of specialised elastic tissues. More of the horse's body is made of muscle than any other tissue. Muscle tissue is bound together in bundles contained within a sheath, often termed a *fascia.* The end of the muscle extends to form a tendon that attaches the muscle to a part of the skeleton.

Muscles need energy to contract and they get this from respiration. Muscles must have a good blood supply from which they get the food and oxygen they need for respiration. Muscle tissue contains many mitochondria to convert food and oxygen to energy for contraction.

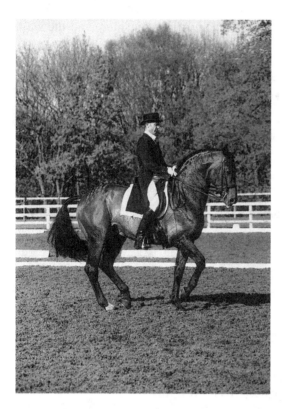

Figure 6.10 Complex manoeuvre of advanced dressage horse.

Functions

Muscles carry out a number of functions:

- Produce movement by contracting
- Help to stabilise joints where two bones meet
- Help to maintain posture
- Help temperature control in the skin by, for example, shivering to gain heat and dilation of skin capillaries for heat loss
- Help give horses their external conformation

Types of muscle

There are three types of muscle:

- *Skeletal* muscle – Includes all muscles attached to bone; also known as *striated* or *voluntary* muscles, as they are under conscious control
- *Smooth* muscle – found in organs such as the bladder and the digestive tract; also known as *involuntary* muscle, as it is not under conscious control
- *Cardiac* muscle – only found in the heart; it makes up the walls of the heart

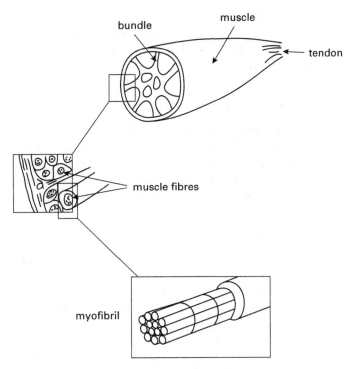

Figure 6.11 Structure of skeletal muscle.

Skeletal, or voluntary, muscle

Skeletal muscle is consciously controlled, for example, the muscles in the limbs which enable the horse to walk, trot, canter, etc. Skeletal muscle consists of muscle fibres made up of tube-shaped cells (Figure 6.11).

Each muscle fibre has a number of nuclei and is enclosed by a sheath known as the *sarcolemma*. These muscle fibres are arranged in bundles lined up in the same direction. Under the microscope they appear to be striped. These stripes, or *striations*, are made up of special proteins, *actin* and *myosin*, which cross the muscle fibre in a crossways or transverse direction giving skeletal muscle the name *striated*. In order for the muscle fibres to contract, the actin filaments slide in between the myosin filaments causing the muscle to become shorter and thicker.

Smooth, or involuntary, muscle

Smooth muscle is not under the horse's conscious control – an example of this type of muscle may be found in the digestive tract, whose muscles contract and relax during peristalsis. Other examples of smooth muscle are found in the walls of blood vessels and in the bladder.

The structure of smooth muscle is different from that of skeletal muscle. The cells are spindle shaped, with one nucleus only. Again, bundles of fibres form a muscle, but under the microscope there are no visible bands or striations.

Cardiac muscle

Cardiac muscle powers the heart and enables it to contract and relax in rhythm throughout the horse's life. It does not become fatigued and does not rely on messages from the brain to make it contract, although the brain may change the rate of contraction of the heart. Cardiac muscle is involuntary and in structure it resembles voluntary muscle.

Skeletal movement

Muscles may be attached via muscle fibres or tendons to each other or to skin, cartilage, ligaments or bone. The moving end of the muscle is known as the *insertion* and the more fixed end, which hardly moves during contraction, is known as the *origin*. Muscle always works in the direction from the origin to the insertion.

Skeletal muscle must pass over a joint to create movement. Most of the horse's body movements use the mechanical principle that states that a force applied to one part of a rigid lever arm is transferred by a pivot point or fulcrum to a weight elsewhere on a lever. In the horse's body, muscles apply force and bones act as the levers with joints being the fulcrums that allow movement to occur.

Contraction of a muscle exerts a pull on part of a bone pulling it towards another bone via its attaching tendon, creating movement. Skeletal muscles do not work alone, but in combination, usually in pairs, and movement usually results from the actions of several pairs of muscles. Each pair of muscles has an *agonist* (contracting muscle) and an *antagonist* (opposing relaxing muscle) that work together to produce a smooth movement.

When a muscle contracts, it does so completely, i.e. muscles cannot partially contract. Involuntary and cardiac muscle contract independently of voluntary control or conscious will. On the other hand, voluntary muscles contract at will, e.g. when the horse lifts its foot for the farrier it does so by intent.

A muscle's ability to keep contracting and relaxing depends upon several factors:

- Available energy
- Time muscle has been contracting
- Blood supply to the muscle
- Temperature of the muscle
- Build-up of lactic acid in the muscle (see Chapter 3, pp. 30–31)

Muscle movement

All muscles contract in order to produce movement, but the type of movement they produce will depend upon their origins and insertions and location within the musculoskeletal system.

The different types of movement are:

- *Flexion* – bend limb
- *Extension* – straighten limb
- *Abduction* – move limb away from the body
- *Adduction* – move limb towards the body
- *Rotation* – head and neck

The horse's superior and deep muscles are shown in Figures 6.12 and 6.13.

Muscle fatigue

Muscles use glycogen/glucose and fatty acids to provide energy for contraction. They burn these energy sources by combining them with

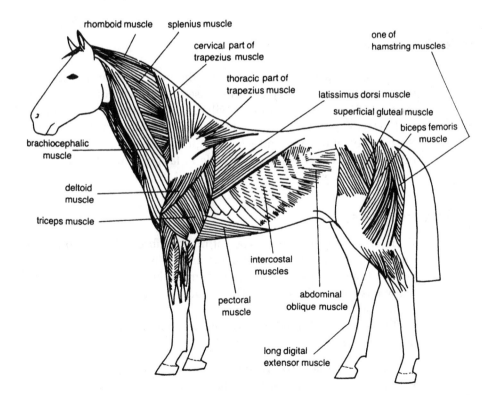

Figure 6.12 Superficial musculature.

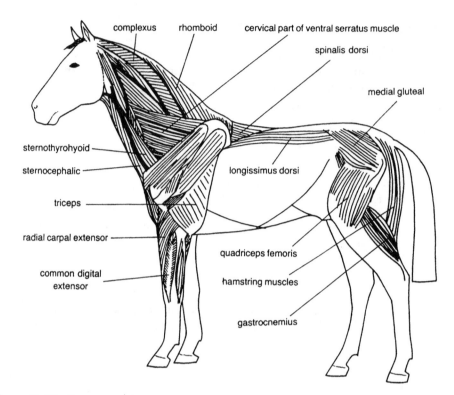

Figure 6.13 Deep musculature.

oxygen from their blood supply. As the muscles continue to work, the heart and respiratory rates increase to provide more oxygen and nutrients. Eventually the muscle will run out of oxygen, and lactic acid will start to build up in the muscle. Eventually this will prevent the muscle contracting and it will begin to tremor (see Oxygen debt, pp. 30–31). At this point the muscle is fatigued and the horse will slow down and stop.

Muscle fibre types

There are several different types of muscle fibre within each muscle. This is exactly the same as in humans, and these fibres have been found when taking small sections of muscle from the living horse, a process known as *biopsy*. These sections are then carefully studied under the microscope.

Muscle can be divided into two groups, depending upon their rates of contraction:

- Slow twitch – slow contraction time
- Fast twitch – fast contraction time

o High oxidative
o Low oxidative

Slow-twitch muscle fibres have a greater ability to use oxygen, which means they can keep contracting at this slower rate for long periods of time. Fast-twitch muscle fibres have fast and powerful contractions. The high-oxidative type can generate power but also has a good ability to use oxygen and can keep working for long periods of time. The slow-oxidative fibres can produce explosive power quickly, but cannot sustain this for long as they can't use as much oxygen and therefore fatigue quickly. These fibres tend to be used for galloping (sprinting) and jumping.

Most muscles consist of a mixture of the three fibre types – slow-twitch and two types of fast-twitch. During muscle contraction it is unlikely that all the muscle fibres will be required to contract all the time in order to produce maximum strength of contraction so there is, in fact, an orderly selection of muscle fibres depending upon the amount of exertion required.

For standing and walking, only slow-twitch muscles are required. As the horse moves faster, fast-twitch high-oxidative fibres are recruited. As the horse accelerates, gallops or jumps, fast-twitch low-oxidative fibres are brought into play. The mixture of fibre types within muscle means a wide range of responses is available to meet the varying demands of the athletic horse.

The proportion of fast-twitch to slow-twitch fibres varies between breeds and types and has a strong genetic component. The Quarter Horse, which is a sprint specialist, has a higher number of fast-twitch fibres than the Arab, a well-known endurance horse. Faster-twitch fibres have a greater diameter in order to generate more power, which results in the bulky muscular physique.

In those horses better suited to long distance work, muscle fibres are thinner, allowing blood vessels carrying oxygen and nutrients to the muscle to reach the fibres easily. This results in a longer, leaner frame.

Thoroughbreds bred for racing have a strong genetic component for sprinting or middle-to-long-distance racing. This relates to the pedigree, one of the main reasons used for selective breeding in racehorses!

Summary points

- Muscles work by contraction of muscle fibres
- Involuntary and cardiac muscles work independently of free will
- Muscles work in pairs, each pair has an agonist and an antagonist
- There are three types of muscle: skeletal, smooth and cardiac
- Horses have three types of fibre within voluntary or skeletal muscle tissue

The Circulation

CARDIOVASCULAR SYSTEM

Horses need a transport system to carry food, oxygen and other essential materials to all the cells in their bodies. This transport system, in all mammals, is the circulatory system, sometimes known as the cardiovascular system. It consists of blood, which carries the essential nutrients in a liquid medium, the blood vessels that carry it and the four-chambered heart, which pumps it around the body so that it reaches all its tissues.

The heart is, in fact, two pumps, running what is often referred to as a *double circulation*. The right side of the heart pumps *deoxygenated* blood (blood that is low in oxygen) to the lungs, where it picks up oxygen from inhaled air. The left side then pumps this *oxygenated* blood (blood that is rich in oxygen) around the horse's body, supplying its cells with essential oxygen and nutrients (Figure 7.1). The blood in the right and left sides of the heart cannot mix, so that oxygenated blood does not merge with deoxygenated blood. The structure of the heart is shown in Figure 7.2.

As a general rule, the vessels that carry blood away from the heart, under high pressure, are known as *arteries*, the most major of which is the *aorta*, whereas the vessels that carry blood back to the heart, are known as *veins*, the most major of which is known as the *vena cava*.

THE HEART

The heart is a hollow organ made almost entirely of muscle (cardiac muscle), giving it the ability to contract and relax and enabling it to act as a pump. The heart of a 16 hh horse would weigh approximately 4 kg (9 lbs). As the horse gets fitter, the heart size may increase to about 12 lbs. An unusually large heart has been associated with great racehorses such as Eclipse and Pharlap.

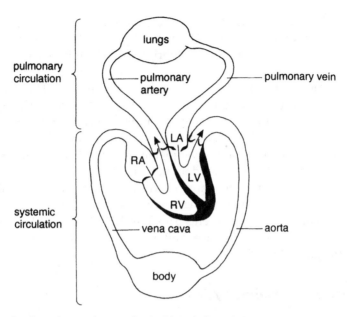

Figure 7.1 Blood circulation, showing the double-sided pump.

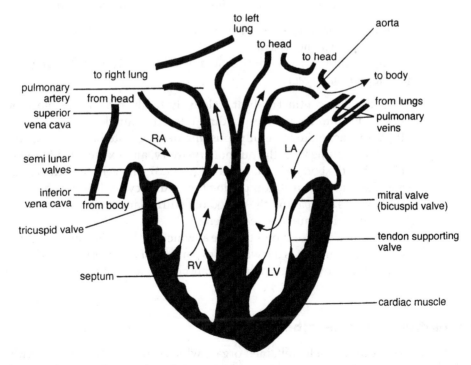

Figure 7.2 Vertical section through the equine heart.

The heart is also surrounded by a membrane known as the *peri-cardium* or *pericardial sac*. This is a completely closed sac, which contains a small amount of fluid for lubrication, which is essential as it allows the heart to move freely as it beats.

The heart is divided into four hollow chambers. The upper two are known as the *atria* and the lower two as the *ventricles*. The right atrium is connected to the right ventricle and the left atrium to the left ventricle by their respective *atrioventricular* openings. It is important to remember that the right side is completely separate from the left side so that blood from the two sides does not mix.

Ventricles are much more powerful and have thicker walls than the atria. Various valves in the heart make sure that blood flows in this direction only and prevents backflow. Blood from the left ventricle has to travel a greater distance to all parts of the horse's body and not just to the lungs, hence the thicker muscular wall.

The cardiac or pumping cycle

The heart is the pump that drives the whole circulatory system; it pushes blood around the body and receives it back afterwards. The heartbeat is the pattern of contraction of the heart, or one cycle of the pump.

The cycle begins when blood flows into the right and left atria:

- Right atrium relaxed – deoxygenated blood flows in from the rest of the body, via the *vena cava*
- Left atrium relaxed – oxygenated blood flows in from the lungs via the *pulmonary vein*

The atria then contract or 'beat', relatively gently, pushing the blood on both sides into their corresponding relaxed ventricles. The ventricles then contract quite forcefully, pushing deoxygenated blood out of the heart to the lungs, via the pulmonary artery, and oxygenated blood to the rest of the body, via the aorta (Figure 7.3). The ventricles than relax and the heart is at rest, completing the cardiac cycle. The period of rest is known as *diastole* and the period of ventricular contraction as *systole*. The two periods are of the same length.

The horse's pulse shows the rate at which the heart is pumping blood around the body. It is the wave of expansion of the artery wall as blood is pushed through it. The pulse can be felt at various points on the horse's body (Figure 7.4).

Regulation of the heartbeat

The heart is a self-contained organ, which can carry on working without the direct intervention of the voluntary or involuntary nervous

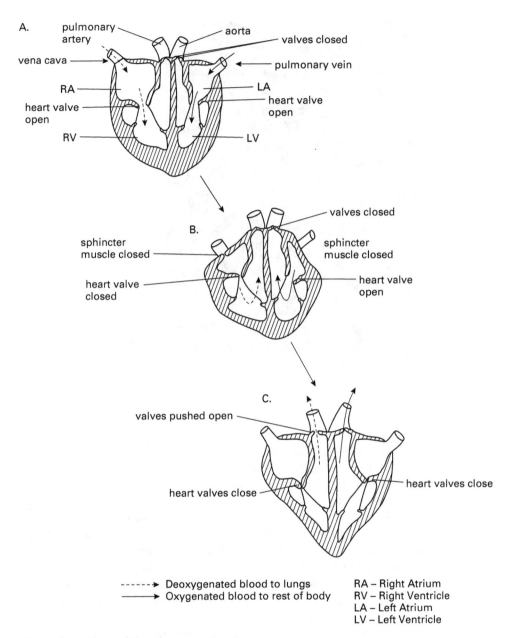

Figure 7.3 The cardiac cycle.

systems. This explains why isolated hearts can continue to beat outside
the body for a long time if kept in the correct environment. The heart
has its own in-built nervous system in the form of a *pacemaker* otherwise known as the *sinoatrial* (SA) node or SAN. The SAN is situated in
the right atrium.

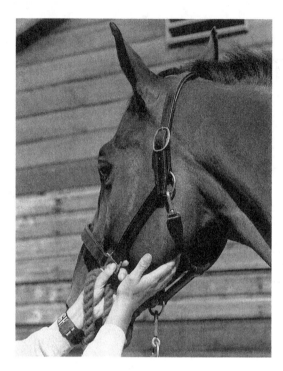

Figure 7.4 Taking the horse's pulse.

The horse's normal resting heartbeat is 36–42 beats per minute. This can be taken using a stethoscope or feeling for the pulse where an artery passes over bone, for example under the jaw (Figure 7.4). When the horse is exercised, the demand for oxygen increases. In order to get this increased oxygen to the cells that require it, the heart has to beat faster to pump the blood to the tissues. The heart of the galloping horse can reach rates of up to 240 beats per minute, at which point it takes only five seconds for a red blood cell to complete one full circuit around the body. By comparison, a human, whose resting heart rate is about 60 beats per minute, can rise to a maximum of only 180 beats per minute.

As shown above, the heart does not always beat at the same rate. Various factors can affect the heart rate:

- Age – faster in foals
- Size of the heart – larger hearts have slower heart rates
- Excitement or fear – adrenaline and nervous stimulation increase the heart rate
- Disease – infection or fever increases the heart rate

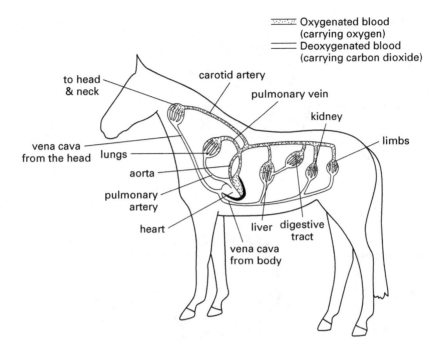

Figure 7.5   The heart and circulation route.

BLOOD VESSELS

There are two main types of blood vessels, *arteries* and *veins*. Most arteries carry oxygenated blood away from the heart and to the rest of the body, and most veins carry deoxygenated blood back to the heart. The exception is the *pulmonary circulation*, in which the *pulmonary artery* carries deoxygenated blood from the heart to the lungs, and the *pulmonary vein* carries oxygenated blood from the lungs to the heart (Figure 7.5). The different characteristics of arteries and veins are summarised in Table 7.1.

Table 7.1   Different characteristics of arteries and veins.

Features of arteries	Features of veins
Take oxygenated blood from the heart	Take deoxygenated blood to the heart
Lumen, or passageway, narrow	Lumen wide
Pumped by heart muscle at high pressure	Pumped by the action of muscles and backflow prevented by valves
Arterial blood contains large amount of nutrients	Venous blood contains a large amount of waste products

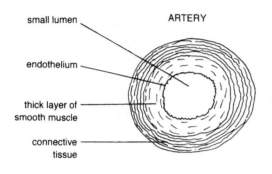

small lumen   ARTERY

endothelium

thick layer of
smooth muscle

connective
tissue

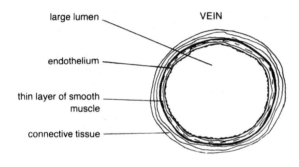

large lumen   VEIN

endothelium

thin layer of smooth
muscle

connective tissue

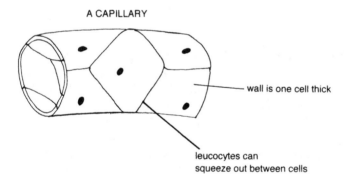

A CAPILLARY

wall is one cell thick

leucocytes can
squeeze out between cells

Figure 7.6 Comparison of
veins and arteries.

Arteries

Blood is carried from the heart to the tissues of the body in vessels
known as arteries. The walls of the arteries are thick and contain muscular and elastic tissue (Figure 7.6). Because it is carrying oxygenated
blood under relatively high pressure, if an artery is cut, bright red blood
will spurt from the wound in time with the heartbeat.

The arteries gradually decrease in size and form branches as they go
further away from the heart. The larger vessels give rise to smaller
ones, which have smooth muscle in their walls. These smaller vessels

are known as *arterioles*, because they are small arteries, still able to contract and regulate blood flow to various organs. The arterioles then become still smaller vessels, called *capillaries*, which they supply with blood. Capillaries are very thin-walled vessels – their walls are only one cell thick. This progressive decrease in artery size is accompanied by a reduction in blood pressure.

At the tissues, the arterial blood gives up its oxygen, nutrients and hormones and collects waste products such as carbon dioxide. The capillaries then converge to form very small veins or *venules* and then progressively larger veins, which carry the deoxygenated blood and its waste products back to the heart.

Veins

Veins have a similar structure to that of arteries, but the walls are much thinner and the proportion of muscular tissue is much less (Figure 7.6). This is because the blood the veins carry, returning to the heart, is under much less pressure. The larger veins contain valves that prevent the backflow of blood. If a vein is cut, dark red, deoxygenated blood will flow from the wound without pulsing.

The small veins, which correspond to the arterioles, are known as *venules*, and also have thin walls. Venules carry deoxygenated blood from the capillaries to the veins. Muscular contractions of the horse's body helps to keep blood moving towards the heart. This is one reason why horses may develop filled legs when standing in a stable for a long time. This forced inactivity inhibits the venous return to the heart and once the horse starts walking again the swelling will often disappear.

Eventually venous blood will enter the great veins or vena cavae and be returned to the right atrium of the heart.

Circulation systems

There are different routes of circulation (Figure 7.5):

- *Systemic* and *portal* circulation
- *Pulmonary* and *coronary* circulation

Systemic circulation

The systemic circulation is the circulation of blood from the heart to the horse's body. Blood is pumped from the heart through the aorta via an extensive network of arteries to the capillaries and body tissues. Blood then returns through a network of veins and eventually to the vena cava and back to the heart.

Portal circulation

The portal circulation supplies the liver from the digestive tract. The veins from the stomach, spleen, pancreas and intestines join together to form the hepatoportal vein taking blood carrying digested nutrients to the liver.

Pulmonary circulation

The pulmonary circulation carries blood from the heart to the lungs and back again. This is the only situation in which an artery carries deoxygenated blood and a vein, oxygenated, i.e. the reverse of the rest of the body.

Deoxygenated blood is taken to the lungs in the pulmonary artery. In the lungs, the blood comes into close contact with the alveoli, and the carbon dioxide it is carrying is exchanged for oxygen by a process known as *gaseous exchange*. In other words, it is oxygenated and then returned to the heart via the pulmonary vein.

Coronary circulation

The coronary circulation supplies the heart muscle with the vital nutrients and oxygen it needs to function. Right and left coronary arteries leave the aorta and supply a network of capillaries that surround the heart. Blood is then returned to the right atrium via the coronary veins.

BLOOD

A type of fluid connective tissue (Chapter 2, pp. 24–5), blood is the body's transport system and consists of a fluid called plasma, in which are suspended red cells, white cells and platelets. There are approximately 7,000,000 red blood cells, 9000 white blood cells and 400,000 platelets per cubic ml of whole blood in horses. Blood consists of 55% plasma and 45% cells. It also carries gases, nutrients, hormones and salts in solution and acts as a communication system, reaching the whole body (Figure 7.7).

Functions

Blood serves a number of functions:

- *Nutrition* – transport of nutrients, also oxygen, enzymes and hormones

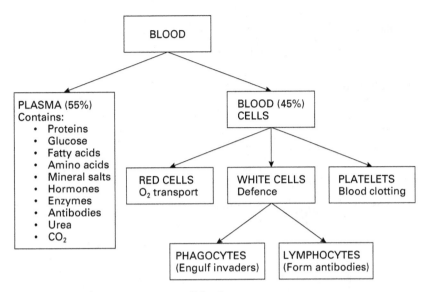

Figure 7.7   The main constituents of blood.

- *Waste disposal* – transport of waste materials, such as carbon dioxide and urea
- *Defence* – transports white cells and antibodies to sites of infection
- *Wound healing* – blood clotting, preventing loss of fluid after injury, transport of healing cells
- *Thermoregulation* – regulation of body temperature

Plasma

Plasma is often referred to as the 'internal environment' which bathes all the cells of the body. It makes up approximately 55% of the blood volume, and about 92% of plasma is water. In addition to water, plasma contains plasma proteins such as albumin, globulin, fibrinogen and prothrombin, and this means that it is slightly thicker than water and is straw coloured. The kidneys are responsible for maintaining a constant level of water and other substances within the plasma.

Other substances dissolved in plasma are:

- Nutrients, such as glucose, glycerol, amino acids, fatty acids, mineral salts, vitamins
- Antibodies
- Hormones
- Enzymes
- Waste products, such as urea and CO_2 (carried mainly as hydrogen carbonate ions)

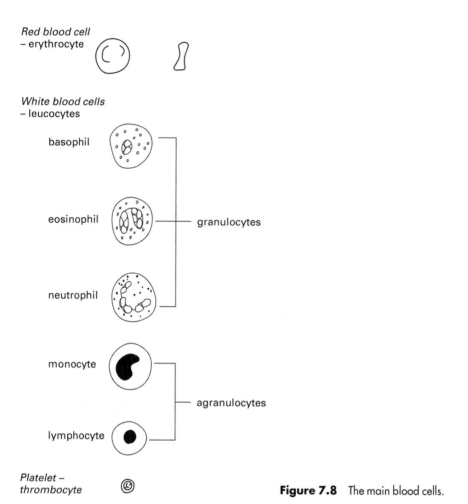

*Red blood cell
– erythrocyte*

*White blood cells
– leucocytes*

basophil

eosinophil — granulocytes

neutrophil

monocyte

agranulocytes

lymphocyte

*Platelet –
thrombocyte*

Figure 7.8   The main blood cells.

Blood cells

There are three types of blood cells: *erythrocytes* (red cells), *leucocytes* (white cells) and *thrombocytes* (platelets). The blood cells of the horse are shown in Figure 7.8.

Red blood cells

Red blood cells are also known as *erythrocytes* or *red corpuscles*. The function of red blood cells is to carry oxygen to all the cells in the horse's body. They are biconcave, or disc-shaped, to give a maximum surface area to carry oxygen. Red blood cells carry oxygen by combining in the lungs with the red pigment *haemoglobin* to form *oxyhaemoglobin* (iron and vitamin B_{12} are also needed). At the body tissues, oxyhaemoglobin gives up the oxygen to nourish them. Red blood cells are unusual in that they do not have a nucleus; this allows more room to carry haemoglobin and therefore oxygen.

It is estimated that horses produce 35 million red blood cells every second of every day. They are made in the red bone marrow within the bone, and have a lifespan of around 120 days. At the end of their usefulness, red blood cells are broken down in the spleen – the iron is then recycled in the liver to prevent loss of this important mineral.

White blood cells

White blood cells are also known as *leucocytes* or *white corpuscles*. These cells have a central role to play in defending the horse's body against disease. White blood cells increase rapidly in number by mitosis in response to disease or injury. They are also larger than red blood cells, have a nucleus and are irregular in shape.

There are two main types of white blood cell or leucocyte:

- *Granulocytes*
- *Agranulocytes* (non-granular leucocytes)

Agranulocytes consist of two types:

- *Phagocytes* (monocytes) – engulf and destroy foreign substances such as bacteria
- *Lymphocytes* – make antibodies, which destroy invading cells; found in all tissues except the brain and spinal cord

Granulocytes make up the majority (75%) of all white blood cells and defend the horse's body against micro-organisms. Granulocytes have the ability to squeeze through capillary walls to enter body tissues to fight off invaders.

Platelets

Platelets, or thrombocytes, are small fragile cells without a nucleus. They are formed in the red bone marrow and are involved in the blood clotting process.

THE LYMPHATIC SYSTEM

The lymphatic system supports the circulatory system and consists of a series of small capillaries, vessels, nodes and ducts containing a fluid known as *lymph*. Blood delivers nutrients and oxygen, etc., to the tissues and collects waste by bathing the tissues in a fluid known as *tissue fluid*. Whole blood itself stays within the blood capillaries. After releasing its nutrients and oxygen and collecting waste products, tissue fluid needs to be returned to the blood. Some of this it can be returned directly to the capillaries, but they are under high pressure. The remainder is collected by the lymphatic capillaries, which are under lower pressure. This fluid is called lymph and makes up 2–3% of the horse's body fluids. The lymphatic capillaries act as a drain for excess tissue fluid, larger molecules, fragments of damaged cells and micro-organisms that may be present.

Lymph is carried to the lymph nodes for filtration before being returned to the bloodstream via the left and right *subclavian veins*. The lymphatic system does not have a pump such as the heart, so how does lymph move from one part of the body to another? There are several methods:

- *Contractions* of skeletal muscles constrict lymphatic vessels, and valves in the vessels prevent lymph going backwards, hence it can only move forwards under contraction
- Negative pressure helps to move the lymph upwards into the lymphatic ducts by *suction*
- Movement of lymph towards the chest area when the horse *inhales*

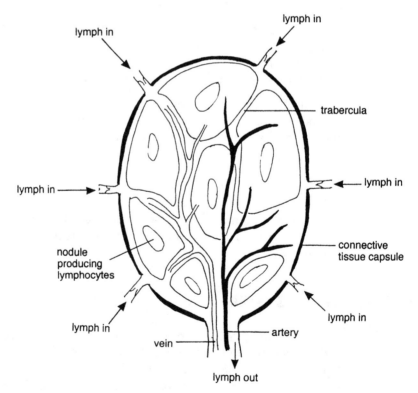

Figure 7.9 Structure of a lymph node.

Obstruction to the flow of lymph will result in its accumulation and hence swelling or *oedema*. This may result in filled legs in horses.

Lymph nodes

All the smaller lymph vessels enter into lymph nodes that are situated throughout the horse's body. The structure of a lymph node is shown in Figure 7.9.

Here the lymph is filtered before returning to the lymphatic system. The function of lymph nodes is to:

- Remove and destroy harmful micro-organisms
- Remove damaged or dead cells
- Remove large protein molecules
- Remove toxic substances
- Produce new lymphocytes and antibodies and add them to lymph where necessary

Lymph nodes swell when there is infection in the area.

Summary points

- The heart is a double pump made of cardiac muscle
- The left side is bigger than the right side
- The left side receives oxygenated blood from the lungs and pumps it around the horse's body
- The right side receives deoxygenated blood from the body and pumps it to the lungs
- Blood carries oxygen and nutrients around the body and collects carbon dioxide and other waste products from the body
- Arteries and veins are the pipe work of the circulatory system
- Red blood cells do not have a nucleus and their function is to carry oxygen around the body
- White blood cells function mainly as a defence against disease
- Platelets are small fragments of cells with a role in blood clotting

---

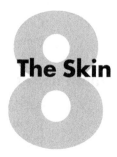

The Skin

The skin is also known as the *integument*. It completely covers the horse's body and therefore is its largest organ. It is water resistant to prevent it becoming waterlogged and also to prevent the loss of valuable fluids from the body.

The skin has many different functions:

- *Defence* – against micro-organisms
- *Protection* – shielding the horse's body from weather
- *Sensory* – sensitive to pain, touch, pressure, heat and cold
- *Thermoregulation* – helps maintain the horse's body temperature
- *Nutrition* – makes vitamin D in the presence of ultraviolet light from the sun
- *Pigmentation* – produces the pigment melanin which gives coat colour
- *Excretion* – excretes urea, a waste product

The structure of the skin is shown in Figure 8.1. There are two layers, known as the *dermis* and *epidermis*. These provide a barrier between the horse and its environment. Skin also varies in thickness depending upon the amount of wear and tear to which it is subject.

STRUCTURE

Epidermis

This is the outer, visible, layer of the skin. It consists of flat, dead skin cells, which are continuously flaking off in a process known as *desquamation*. This layer is often referred to as the *cornified layer*. Cells are replaced from the lower layers of the epidermis. The bottom, *basal layer* produces cells that move gradually higher towards the surface. As they do so, they fill with the protein keratin, flatten and die off. The dead

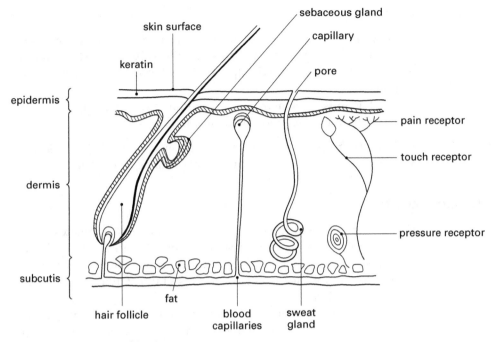

Figure 8.1   Structure of the skin.

layer of cells at the skin's surface is relatively hard and has a protective effect.

The epidermis is also folded inwards in many places to form hair follicles. A hair, made of keratin, grows from each follicle.

The basal layer is also known as the *stratum germinativum* and this layer also contains the skin pigment *melanin*, which gives the skin its natural colour. Cells known as *melanocytes* make melanin.

Dermis

The dermis contains blood and nervous supplies. It is made of connective tissue and is elastic and quite tough. It contains *collagen*, which helps to plump up the skin, and *elastin*, which keeps it supple. Beneath the dermis is a layer of subcutaneous fat, which helps to insulate the horse's body from the cold and also acts as an energy store.

The dermis has several functions:

- Contains sweat glands which help in temperature regulation
- Contains blood vessels which bring nourishment to and take waste products from the skin and help with temperature regulation
- Contains nerve endings sensitive to touch, pressure, pain, temperature

Glands

The dermis contains *sebaceous* glands, which are attached to each hair follicle (Figure 8.1). These produce an oily substance, *sebum*, which lubricates the hair shaft and helps keep the skin supple and resistant to wetting.

Sweat glands stretch from deep within the dermis layer to the surface. There are two kinds of sweat glands:

- *Apocrine* – respond to nervous stimulation, resulting in frothy sweat
- *Eccrine* – secrete watery sweat for rapid cooling by evaporation

Hair and coat

Hair is a structure of the epidermis, even though it originates in the dermis, which is made up of dead cells containing keratin. Each hair has a shaft, set at an angle to the skin, and a root, which lies within the base of the hair follicle. At its base, there is a bulb of living tissue where growth takes place.

The horse has a thick coat in winter and a light coat in summer (Figures 8.2 and 8.3). The temporary hair is shed every spring and autumn in response to metabolic and hormonal changes that are triggered by changing day length and environmental temperature.

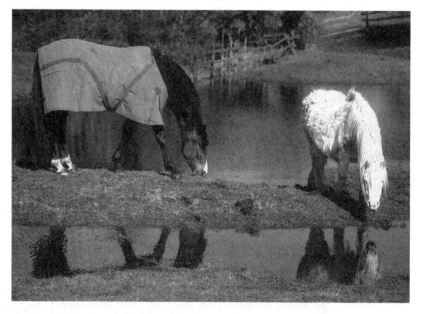

Figure 8.2 Pony with thick, woolly, winter coat.

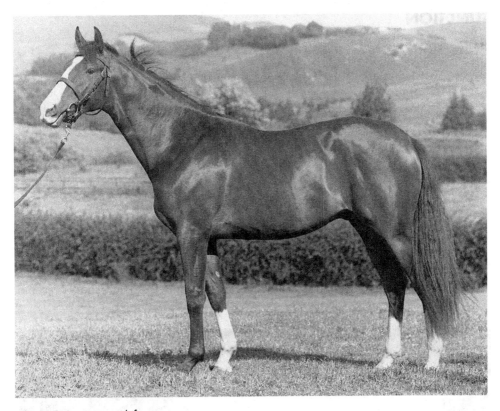

Figure 8.3   Horse with fine summer coat.

The horse's skin carries several different types of hair:

- *Permanent* hair – tail, mane, eyelashes, feathers
- *Tactile* hair – whiskers of the muzzle
- *Temporary* hair – makes up the bulk of the coat

The temporary hair consists of longer hairs, which cover a dense undercoat of tightly-packed shorter hairs.

Coat colour

Skin and coat colour depend upon the presence of a pigment called *melanin*. Pigment cells in the epidermis called *melanocytes* produce melanin. Horses have two types of pigment:

- *Eumelanin* – black/brown
- *Phaeomelanin* – red/yellow

This pigment is produced under genetic control, which makes coat colour a genetically determined variable.

FUNCTION

Protection

The skin protects against micro-organisms, not only by acting as a physical barrier, but also because of its pH. The pH of the skin is naturally acidic and this inhibits the growth of micro-organisms.

Melanin also helps protect the skin from the harmful fraction of ultraviolet rays from the sun.

Nutrition

Vitamin D, a vitamin that is essential for the maintenance of healthy bone, is made in the skin. Vitamin D is taken to body tissues via the blood and any excess is stored in the liver. It is made from a substance in the skin called *ergosterol*, in the presence of ultraviolet light. Horses kept stabled all year round, or those kept out with rugs on all year (Figure 8.4), will not produce enough vitamin D, so they should receive dietary supplementation.

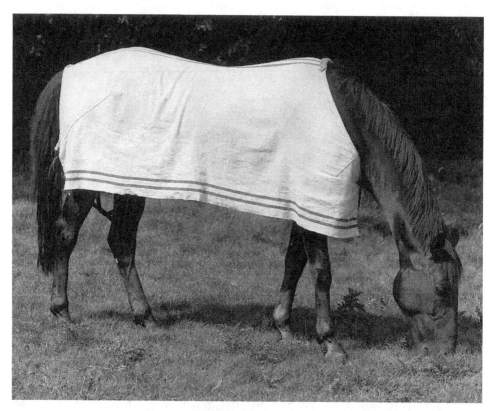

Figure 8.4 Horses that are turned out with rugs on may need vitamin D supplementation.

Heat production and loss

A constant balance must be maintained between heat produced in the horse's body and heat lost to or gained from the environment. Most of the heat lost from the horse's body is from the surface. Some heat is also lost via the urine, faeces and exhaled air.

Mechanisms of heat loss include:

- *Conduction* – rugs and any other objects in direct contact with the horse's skin take up heat
- *Convection* – air that passes over a horse's body is heated by the skin and rises, to be replaced by cooler air; heat is also lost in this way by the rugs worn by the horse
- *Radiation* – all parts of the horse's body that are not covered by rugs etc. radiate heat away from the body

Energy, in the form of heat, is released within cells during metabolic reactions, so that the most active organs will produce the most heat:

- *Muscles* – horses have large muscle masses – the harder the muscles work, the more heat is produced; when the horse's body temperature falls, it shivers in order to produce warmth
- *Liver* – a chemically active organ which produces heat
- *Digestive system* – heat is produced by chemical reactions involved both in digestion and peristalsis

Thermoregulation – temperature control

To maintain the horse's body temperature at a constant level, the skin and other parts of the body work together under the control of a part of the brain known as the *hypothalamus*. The hypothalamus detects the temperature of blood flowing through it, and, if it varies from the normal, it sends messages, via the nervous system, to the different parts of the body connected with maintaining body temperature, or *thermoregulation*.

Fall in body temperature

If the body temperature falls, the hypothalamus sends messages that cause the body to respond in a number of ways (Figure 8.5):

- *Shivering* – muscles in the body contract and relax quickly to produce heat
- *Hair* – the erector muscles in the skin contract, pulling the hairs so that they stand up, trapping an insulating layer of air in the horse's coat that helps to reduce heat loss from the body

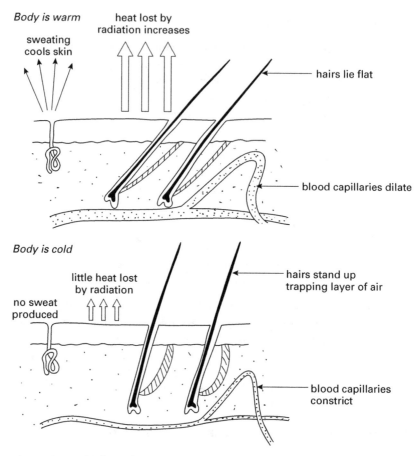

Figure 8.5   The skin aids temperature regulation.

- *Blood circulation* – capillaries just below the skin surface contract, pushing blood through the deeper capillaries to help reduce heat loss from the skin
- *Respiration* – metabolic activity in the liver increases, breaking down more glucose to produce heat and warming the blood, which carries this heat around the body

Rise in body temperature

The hypothalamus detects a rise in blood temperature and sends messages via the nervous system resulting in the following effects (Figure 8.5):

- *Blood circulation* – capillaries near the skin surface dilate, or widen, taking more blood to the surface, which this helps to cool the blood by transfer of heat to the air by radiation

- *Respiration* – metabolic activity in the liver reduces so less heat is produced
- *Hair* – the erector muscles in the skin relax, allowing hair to lie flat so little air is trapped and the insulation effect is minimal
- *Sweat* – the sweat glands secrete sweat which evaporates from the skin, producing a cooling effect

Sweat

Like hairs, sweat glands are epidermal structures even though they extend into the dermis. A sweat gland consists of a coiled tube that opens onto the skin surface. When the horse's body temperature and/or the external ambient temperature increase, adrenalin stimulates the sweat glands to produce sweat.

Horses are able to sweat freely everywhere except the legs. Some areas in particular, such as behind the ears, the flanks and over the neck, contain large numbers of sweat glands. Heat is lost as sweat evaporates from the surface of the skin producing a cooling effect. Horses may be seen to be sweating with excitement at the start of a race (Figure 8.6).

Sweating is a continuous process, but sweat is only visible on the surface of the skin when the rate of sweating is greater than the evaporation rate, when a horse's skin starts to become wet with sweat.

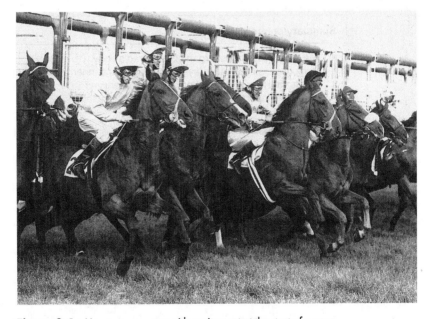

Figure 8.6 Horses may sweat with excitement at the start of a race.

A horse grazing in the heat of a summer's day may lose as much as six litres of fluid per day, without any visible wetness of the coat.

Sweating is influenced by many factors, including:

- Environmental temperature
- Humidity – moisture in the air reduces the horse's ability to lose sweat by evaporation, so effective heat loss is reduced
- Length of coat
- Level of work
- Degree of fitness
- Insulation by fat (depth of fat under the skin)
- Excitement, fear, raised body temperature, pain

The actual ambient temperature and the degree of humidity are used to produce a figure for the *effective temperature*. The combination of high ambient temperature and high relative humidity will produce a high effective temperature and will reduce the horse's ability to sweat effectively. This can result in severe problems with heat exhaustion for horses competing in hot and humid climates.

Horse sweat is hypertonic, that is it contains a higher concentration of mineral salts than in the horse's blood. This means they may lose body salts very quickly when they sweat profusely, and these mineral salts, or electrolytes, must be replaced in the diet. Horses also lose protein in sweat, which gives the frothy, lathered appearance.

Summary points

- The skin is the largest organ of the horse's body
- Skin consists of an outer layer (epidermis) and inner layer (dermis)
- Skin is vital for protection from harmful organisms
- Skin is an important organ for temperature regulation

The Respiratory System

Breathing is the process by which horses gain oxygen from the air and remove carbon dioxide from the body. Air that is breathed in is known as *inhaled* air whereas that which is breathed out is known as *exhaled* air. Exhaled air contains more carbon dioxide and less oxygen than inhaled air.

As the horse breathes in, air is drawn into the lungs, where oxygen is taken into the blood and circulated around the body for cellular respiration. The carbon dioxide that is produced as a waste product of this cellular respiration is then added to the blood, taken to the lungs and breathed out.

The exchange of oxygen and carbon dioxide in the lungs is known as *gaseous exchange*, and this is discussed later in this chapter.

The functions of the respiratory system include:

- Provision of oxygen to the body
- Removal of carbon dioxide from the body
- Temperature control (breathing out warm air, taking in cool air)
- Communication (through the vocal cords)
- Sense of smell and touch (sensory hairs on the nose)
- Filter out air-borne invaders

The respiratory system of the horse is shown in Figure 9.1. The lungs are divided into left and right sides, and these are subdivided into lobes. They are situated in the chest, or *thorax*, and the sides of the chest are constrained by the ribs. Between the ribs are the *intercostal* muscles. Behind the lungs is a dome-shaped sheet of muscle tissue, the *diaphragm*, which separates the chest from the abdomen. Two thin sheets of tissue, the *pleural membranes*, with a thin layer of fluid between them, surround the lungs. This fluid is important as it acts as a lubricant, allowing membranes to slide smoothly as lung movement during breathing takes place.

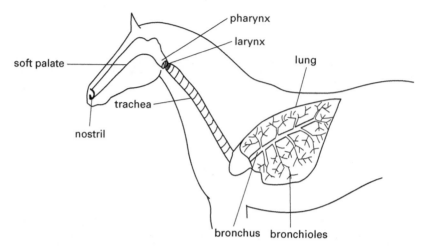

Figure 9.1   The respiratory system.

PARTS OF THE RESPIRATORY SYSTEM

Nose

As horses inhale, air is drawn deep into the lungs, the main organs of the respiratory system. Horses cannot breathe through their mouths as can humans, but draw air in through their nostrils into the two nasal cavities continuous with each nostril. The nasal cavities are separated from each other by a piece of cartilage, and from the mouth by the hard and soft palates. Each side of the nasal cavity is partly filled with three wafer-thin bones called *turbinate* bones. These are curled to increase their surface area. At the front of the skull are large air-filled cavities known as sinuses and these are also connected to the nasal cavity. The airways of the head are shown in Figure 9.2.

The nasal cavity and turbinate bones are lined by a mucous membrane, which helps to warm, moisten and clean inhaled air. The mucous membranes are lined with ciliated epithelium, which is covered with tiny hair-like projections called *cilia*. Dust and germs get caught up in the mucus produced by the mucous membrane, and the cilia move in waves, pushing mucus and debris to the throat where it is either swallowed or coughed up (Figure 9.3). The mucous membrane lining also contains the olfactory nerves associated with the horse's sense of smell (see Chapter 10, pp. 131–2).

The functions of the nose include:

- *Moistening* and *warming* inhaled air
- Sense of smell
- *Filtering* dust, bacteria and foreign material from the inhaled air

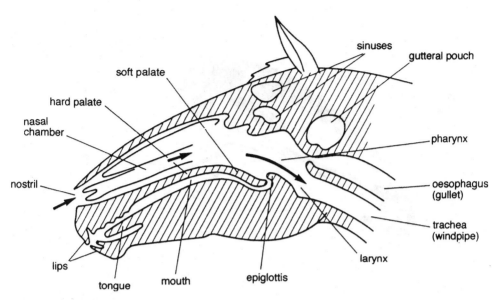

Figure 9.2 Airways of the horse's head.

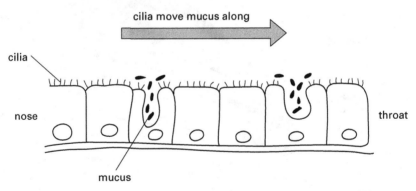

Figure 9.3 Airway cilia.

Pharynx (throat)

The pharynx is a tube leading from the back of the nose and mouth (Figure 9.4). It divides into the *oesophagus*, which carries food to the stomach, and the *trachea*, which takes air to the lungs. The oesophagus lies above and behind the trachea.

The *Eustachian tubes* have outlets at the top of the pharynx, allowing air to enter the middle ear, and they are also connected to the *guttural pouches* that lie just above the pharynx.

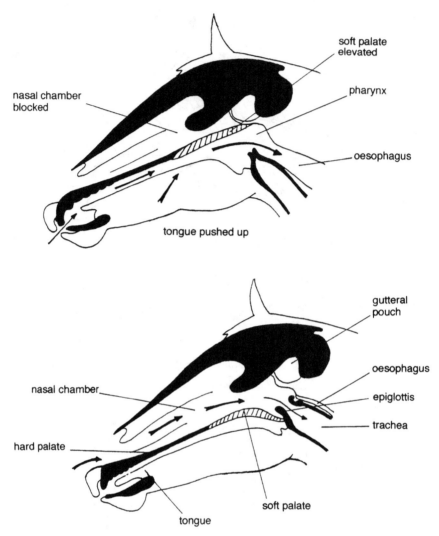

Figure 9.4 The pharynx.

Larynx

The larynx is a short tube-like structure, which is sited between the pharynx and trachea. It is also known as the *voice box* as it houses the vocal chords that enable sound to be produced (the horse can neigh, whinny, moan and nicker). The most important functions of the larynx are to control the flow of air during breathing and prevent foreign material, such as food and other debris, from entering the trachea.

The larynx is made up of five rings of cartilage attached to one another by ligaments and membranes. These cartilage rings also serve as attachments for muscles, which open and close the opening of the larynx, the *glottis*. The muscles also close the lid of the larynx (*epiglottis*) when the horse is swallowing, thereby preventing food from entering the airways.

The larynx filters dust and bacteria from the air, however some dust will enter the trachea if the horse is in a dusty environment.

Trachea (windpipe)

The trachea is a continuation of the larynx and leads to the chest (*thorax*) where it divides into two smaller airways, or *bronchi*. It is easily felt running along the lower border of the horse's neck.

The trachea is made up of 48–60 incomplete rings of hyaline cartilage, which help to keep this part of the airway open at all times. The trachea is lined with mucus-secreting cells, which secrete sticky mucus that traps any foreign material that enters the trachea. This is then wafted back up the windpipe by cilia.

Lungs

The structure of the horse's lung is shown in Figure 9.5.

Bronchi (singular: bronchus)

The trachea divides into two bronchi just above the heart, one branch going into each lung. The two bronchi then divide and divide again to form smaller *bronchioles*. The bronchi are the branches of the respiratory tube which transport air into and out of each lung and they are also made of hyaline cartilage.

Bronchioles

The last and finest tubes of the airways, bronchioles are made of fibrous and elastic tissue. They become progressively smaller as they spread deeper into the lungs until they are no more than a single layer of epithelial cells thick. Bronchioles take air to the *alveoli*.

Alveoli

The alveoli are tiny blind-ending sacs situated at the ends of the bronchioles. Alveoli (singular: *alveolus*) are made of a thin layer of squamous epithelial cells and are surrounded by a blood capillary network. The function of the alveoli is *gaseous exchange*.

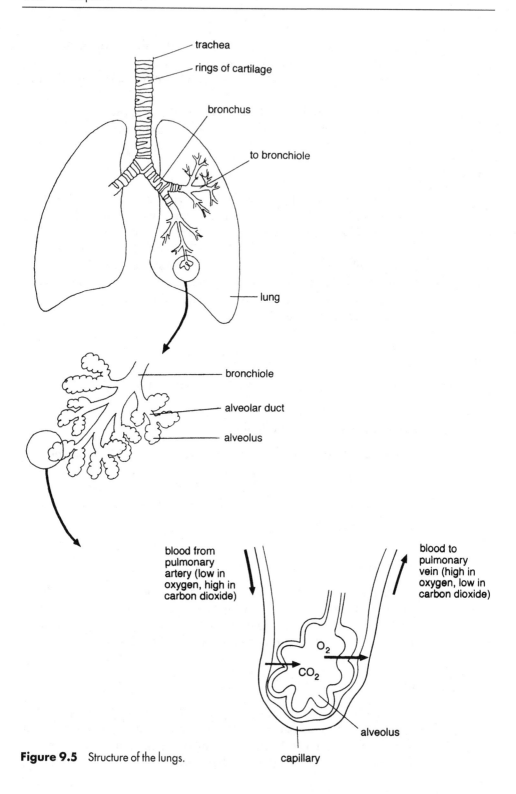

trachea

rings of cartilage

bronchus

to bronchiole

lung

bronchiole

alveolar duct

alveolus

blood from pulmonary artery (low in oxygen, high in carbon dioxide)

blood to pulmonary vein (high in oxygen, low in carbon dioxide)

O₂

CO₂

alveolus

capillary

Figure 9.5   Structure of the lungs.

PHYSICAL MECHANISMS OF RESPIRATION

Gaseous exchange

The term *gaseous exchange* refers to the important exchange of gases between the alveoli and the blood. This process takes place following the rules of an important law of physics which states that 'Gases diffuse from an area of higher pressure to a lower pressure until equal pressure is achieved.' This means that gases will diffuse if a strong concentration of gas comes into contact with a weak concentration of the same gas (see Chapter 1, pp. 13–14). The gas will diffuse into the area of low concentration until balance has been achieved, and this is the physical basis for gaseous exchange.

In the alveoli, air breathed in is rich in oxygen, and the blood (which has returned from giving up its oxygen to the rest of the body) is now low in oxygen. Oxygen then passes from the air in the alveoli to the blood capillaries (Figure 9.6). At the same time, carbon dioxide (picked up as a waste product of cellular respiration) from the blood is at a high level and this passes into the alveoli to be breathed out. This occurs until the concentration of both gases is equal on both sides. The blood is then taken to the left side of the heart before being pumped around the

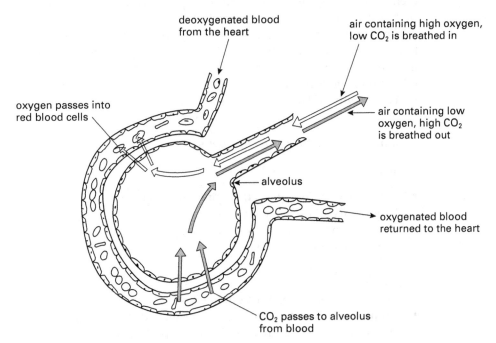

Figure 9.6   *Gaseous exchange in an alveolus.*

horse's body. (See Chapter 7, pp. 84–92, for a detailed discussion of the pulmonary circulation.) When blood reaches the tissues, oxygen is passed to the cells by the same method and carbon dioxide collected. Cells that work harder, such as muscle cells, will pick up more oxygen and release more carbon dioxide.

Breathing

Air enters the horse's body through the same gaseous pressure principle: the pressure in the lungs is lower than the air pressure outside of the body. But the action of muscles within the horse's chest makes this possible. The main muscle involved is the *diaphragm*, which is aided by the *intercostal* muscles that lie between the ribs.

The diaphragm is a large muscle, which separates the chest and abdomen. It is made of a central sheet of tendon with muscle fibres attached at the edges. When relaxed, the diaphragm has a dome shape, with the rounded part of the dome towards the lungs, and when it contracts it flattens out. It contracts during *inhalation* (breathing in), drawing air into the lungs, and relaxes during *exhalation* (breathing out). When it relaxes, it regains its dome shape, which pushes into the chest cavity, making the cavity smaller and thereby increasing the pressure within it. Because the pressure is now lower outside, the air then rushes out. (The diaphragm also helps with other body processes, such as urination, defecation and birth.)

The intercostal muscles aid the diaphragm by contracting at the same time as the diaphragm, lifting the rib cage out and up, thereby increasing the size of the chest cavity during inhalation. This is followed by relaxation of these muscles and the diaphragm, reducing the volume of the chest cavity and causing exhalation (Figure 9.7).

Summary of breathing mechanisms

Inhalation:

- Intercostal muscles contract, moving ribs up and out
- Diaphragm contracts and flattens
- Volume of the chest increases, reducing pressure
- Air is drawn into the lungs

Exhalation:

- Intercostal muscles relax, ribs move down and in
- Diaphragm relaxes and becomes dome-shaped, moving up
- Volume of the chest decreases, increasing pressure
- Air is forced out of the lungs

Breathing in

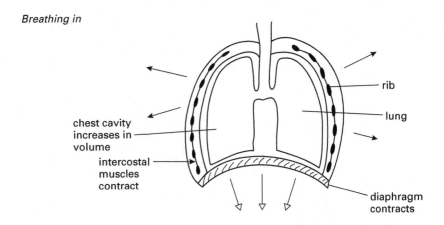

chest cavity
increases in
volume

rib

lung

intercostal
muscles
contract

diaphragm
contracts

Breathing out

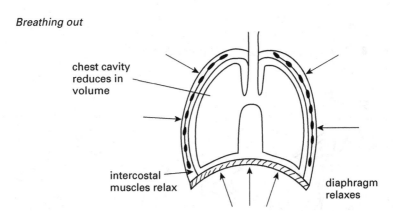

chest cavity
reduces in
volume

intercostal
muscles relax

diaphragm
relaxes

Figure 9.7   Breathing movement of the chest.

A comparison of the different compositions of gases in inhaled and
exhaled air is shown in Figure 9.8.

Breathing rate

The normal resting breathing rate of the horse is 8–16 breaths per
minute. Exercise may increase this to 120 breaths per minute. The horse
is unusual in that the rate of breathing is linked to the horse's gait.
At gallop, the stride rate equals the respiration rate. This means the
muscles of breathing and movement do not work against each other.
As the galloping horse lifts its legs, the head is raised, the gut moves
back and the horse breathes in. As the horse lands, the head drops, the
gut moves forward and the horse breathes out (Figure 9.9).

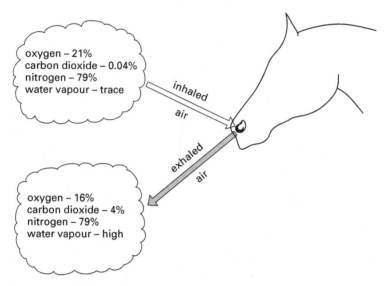

Figure 9.8 Composition of gases in inhaled and exhaled air.

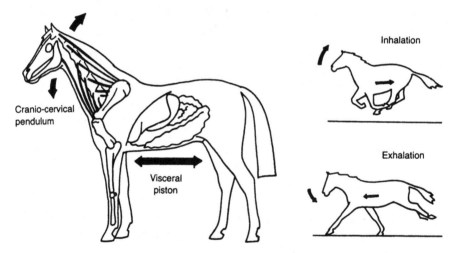

Figure 9.9 Movement in relation to inhalation/exhalation.

Summary points

- Breathing enables horses to gain oxygen and remove carbon dioxide from the body
- Breathing helps in temperature control
- The respiratory system is vital for gaseous exchange
- Ciliated epithelial cells produce mucus to trap debris
- The horse's breathing rate is linked to its gait

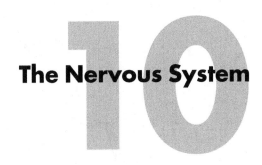

The Nervous System

In order to survive, horses need fast and efficient internal communication systems with which to respond to their environment. They have two co-ordinating systems, the *endocrine* (hormonal) and *nervous* systems that work together triggering responses to their environment. The flight or fight response to danger is brought about by both nervous and hormonal signals, however the nervous system response is much faster.

The main differences between the nervous and endocrine systems are:

Table 10.1 A comparison of the horse's nervous and endocrine systems.

Nervous system	Endocrine system
Messages rapid	Messages slow
Messages go to specific points	Messages go to all parts of the body via the bloodstream
Responses usually localised	Responses may be widespread
Responses short-lived	Responses may continue for long periods

For convenience, the nervous system is divided into two main parts:

- Central nervous system (CNS) – the brain and spinal cord
- Peripheral nervous system (PNS) – mostly communication nerves, which carry signals from the CNS to the rest of the body

NERVE CELLS (NEURONS)

Nervous tissue is composed of:

- Nerve cells, or *neurons*, with attached fibres
- *Neuroglia* – specialised connective tissue that supports the neurons but does not transmit messages

Nerve cells are the basic unit of the nervous system. They are elongated and narrow and may be up to 1 m long. Unlike other cells in the horse's

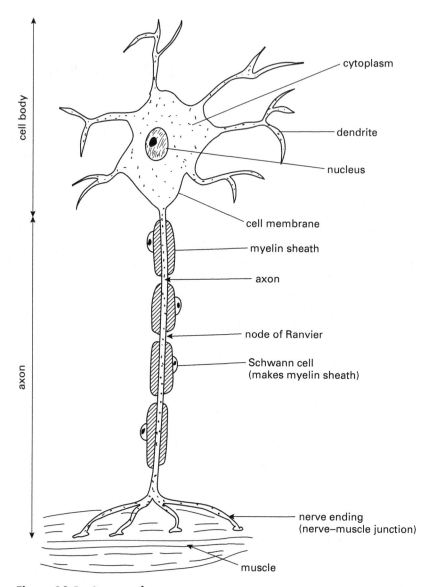

cytoplasm

dendrite

nucleus

cell membrane

myelin sheath

axon

node of Ranvier

Schwann cell
(makes myelin sheath)

nerve ending
(nerve–muscle junction)

muscle

cell body

axon

Figure 10.1 Structure of a neuron.

body, they are not normally replaced when they die, although current research suggests that some may have the ability to regenerate.

The structure of a typical neuron is shown in Figure 10.1; however, depending upon their specific function and location in the body, their shape and size vary (Figure 10.2). The three main types of neuron are:

- Unipolar
- Bipolar
- Multipolar

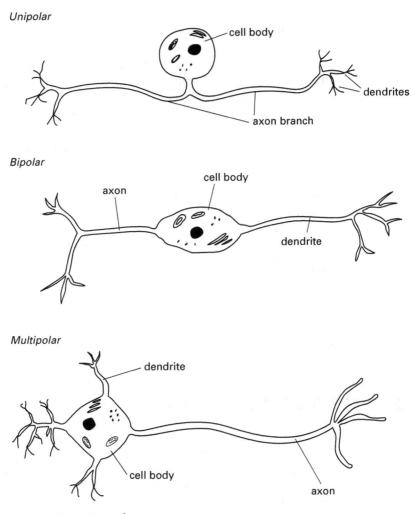

Unipolar

cell body

dendrites

axon branch

Bipolar

cell body

axon

dendrite

Multipolar

dendrite

cell body

axon

Figure 10.2 Types of neuron.

Neurons act as a chain, passing information from one to the next until they reach their target. The neurones do not touch, although the axon of one is close to the dendrite of another; messages actually jump across the gap or *synapse* via specialised chemicals known as *neurotransmitters*. These are released by the nerve endings. The functions of the different parts of the neuron are as follows:

- *Cell body* – centre of the neuron; contains the nucleus and cytoplasm (see Chapter 2, pp. 17–19)
- *Dendrites* – these are nerve fibres often branched, which transmit nerve impulses to the cell body; most neurons have several dendrites
- *Axon* – a single long fibre that transmits nerve impulses away from the cell body; most neurons have only one axon

- *Myelin sheath* – a sheath made of a fatty substance, myelin, that covers the axon; acts as an insulator, protecting the axon and helping to increase the speed conduction of nerve impulses
- *Neurilemma* – A delicate membrane that surrounds the axon and helps regenerate nerve cells; found only in peripheral nerves and not those of the brain or spinal cord
- *Nodes of Ranvier* – compressed indents in the myelin sheath; these help to speed up nerve impulses
- *Axon terminals* – Pass on nerve impulses to the dendrites of the next neuron in the chain
- *Synapse* – small gap between two neurons where they meet; filled with a neurotransmitter that transfers the nerve impulse from one neuron to the other

Although individual neurons have a common structure and function, they are arranged to make up five different types of nerves within the horse's body:

(1) Motor (efferent) nerves
(2) Sensory (afferent) nerves
(3) Mixed – both motor and sensory
(4) White matter
(5) Grey matter

CENTRAL NERVOUS SYSTEM (CNS)

The horse's nervous system detects and interprets changes in conditions both inside and outside the horse's body, and then responds to them, helping to protect it from harm. The environmental change, or *stimulus*, is first received and then conducted to a central control system, which interprets the message and causes appropriate action to be taken. The control system is known as the central nervous system and consists of the brain and spinal cord, which are protected by the skull and spinal column respectively.

The brain is the main unit and is connected to the rest of the horse's body by nerve cells that act as messengers, carrying information to and instructions from the brain. The CNS receives input from the sense organs, such as the skin, eyes, ears, etc., and sends signals to the muscles and glands via the peripheral nervous system.

Brain

The horse's brain is relatively small compared to its body size, weighing around 0.65 kg (1.5 lb), which equates to about 1% of its body weight. The human brain, for comparison, weighs 1.3 kg (3 lb). The brain is the control

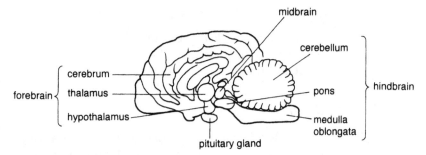

Figure 10.3 Structure of the brain.

centre of the nervous system. It fills the horse's skull and is made up of millions of highly-organised neurons. The brain has a jelly-like consistency and is protected by layers of membranes known as the *meninges*. The skull and meninges together help to protect the brain from damage.

The brain has three different sections (Figure 10.3):

- Cerebrum
- Cerebellum
- Brain stem

Cerebrum

The cerebrum is much smaller than that in the human brain. The horse is not considered to be a highly intelligent animal, but rather an animal of instinct, and this shows in its behaviour. The cerebrum is folded to increase surface area, so that it can accommodate more neurons. It is the largest and most sophisticated part of the horse's brain and is divided into left and right cerebral hemispheres.

The outer layer is made up of folds of grey matter. These are cell bodies of the neurons. Inside the grey matter is the white matter, which consists of the fibres of the neurons. The nerve fibres connect different parts of the brain.

The cerebrum has the following functions:

- Control of voluntary movement
- Reaction to sensation such as heat, cold, touch, smell, sight, etc.
- Control of memory and reasoning

Cerebellum

The cerebellum is situated below the cerebrum and above the medulla oblongata. It also consists of two hemispheres, both filled with grey matter, with white matter within.

The cerebellum has the following functions:

- Co-ordinates muscle movement so it is smooth and not jerky
- Maintains co-ordination and balance
- Maintains muscle tone and shape

Brain stem

The brain stem is made up of three parts, known as the *medulla oblongata, midbrain* and *pons varolii*. The midbrain and *pons varolii* transmit messages to and from the spinal cord, cerebrum and cerebellum, acting as relay centres.

The *medulla oblongata* is the lowest part of the brain stem. It has white matter on the surface and grey matter within, i.e. the opposite of the cerebellum and cerebrum. It is a vital part of the brain, as it is responsible for controlling the cardiovascular and respiratory systems. Functions of the medulla oblongata include:

- Controls rate and force of contraction of the heart
- Controls rate and depth of breathing
- Controls constriction and dilation of blood vessels
- Is the reflex centre, controlling coughing, sneezing and swallowing

Hypothalamus

The *hypothalamus* is a part of the brain about the size of a cherry. It sits just below the midbrain and actually forms part of the base of this part of the brain. Although not itself an endocrine gland, it exerts control over many of the endocrine glands including the thyroid, adrenals, ovaries and testes (see Chapter 11, pp. 134–5). It is essential for regulating metabolism, temperature and water balance and is the centre of autonomic nervous activity (see below). It creates thirst, hunger and pain. The hypothalamus is also responsible for regulation of the pituitary gland.

Spinal cord

The spinal cord extends from the medulla oblongata to the end of the horse's tail vertebrae. There are more than ten billion nerve cells within the spinal cord, and it is housed within the horse's spine. The spinal cord has white matter on the surface and grey matter within. Sprouting from the spinal cord on each side at regular intervals are pairs of spinal nerves.

The spinal cord carries both sensory and motor nerve fibres, which send messages to and from the brain to the horse's body, along its length.

PERIPHERAL NERVOUS SYSTEM (PNS)

The PNS consists of all the nerves that connect the brain and spinal cord to the rest of the horse's body, including the cranial and spinal nerves. The nerves that carry signals to and from the brain are known as *cranial nerves*, whereas those that carry signals to and from the spinal cord are known as the *spinal* nerves. The horse's eyes, nose, tongue and ears, for example, are served by the cranial nerves, whereas the muscles and skin of the legs are serviced by the spinal nerves.

Hundreds of thousands of signals both incoming and outgoing, pass each other within the same nerves all the time.

AUTONOMIC NERVOUS SYSTEM (ANS)

The autonomic nervous system is responsible for controlling most of the horse's internal organs, such as the intestines, lungs and liver. It consists of two systems of neurons that have opposing effects on most of the internal organs. One set, the *parasympathetic* system, prepares the body for activities which gain and conserve energy in the body such as stimulation of the salivary glands and digestive juices and decreasing of the heart and respiratory rates. The other set of neurons, known as the *sympathetic* system, has the opposite effect, preparing the horse's body for energy consuming activities such as fight or flight: the digestive organs are slowed down, the heart and respiratory rates are increased and the liver releases glucose into the blood.

Both the CNS and the PNS contribute to the ANS.

REFLEXES

Reflexes are a small but important part of the behaviour of horses, and largely serve protective functions. A reflex is an action that occurs automatically and immediately and, more importantly, predictably, to a particular external stimulus. This reflex action is completely independent of the will of the horse, i.e. it is governed by the ANS so the horse cannot control the action voluntarily.

The simplest reflex action would be perhaps the horse's skin responding to pressure or heat. A sensory nerve cell or neuron is stimulated by heat. It sends an impulse along its axon or nerve fibre to the CNS. Here the fibre connects to a motor-nerve cell, or neuron, which stimulates the muscle to move the horse away from the heat. This pattern is known as a *reflex arc* (Figure 10.4). Most reflex arcs are more complicated than this example, however.

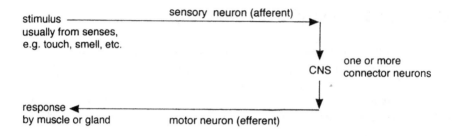

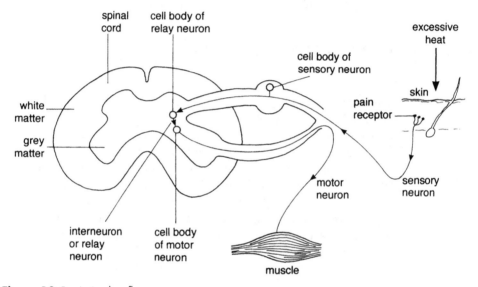

Figure 10.4 A simple reflex arc.

Many reflexes, such as shivering in response to cold or emptying the bladder when it is full, are present from birth. Examples of reflex actions include:

- Shivering
- Urinating
- Sneezing
- Coughing
- Swallowing
- Blinking

The horse is able to sleep standing up due to a postural reflex action.

Conditioned reflexes

Other reflexes are conditioned, in that they are learned by the horse through experiences during its lifetime. These experiences result in the formation of new pathways and junctions within the nervous system itself. The way in which these processes are acquired is known as *conditioning*. Learning is a type of conditioning in that once a response to a new situation has been repeated several times, then a response becomes automatically initiated next time that stimulus occurs. For example, a horse will learn to move away from the handler when a hand is placed against his side. Eventually, this will be done automatically and without conscious will.

THE SENSES

Like all mammals, horses have specialised organs that help to give them an awareness of their environment. These are essential for survival. There are sense organs responsible for sight, hearing (and balance), smell and taste. They are all extensions of the brain and are directly connected to it by nerves. These special sense organs differ tremendously from each other in both structure and function. The senses of the horse are:

- Sight
- Hearing
- Smell
- Taste
- Touch

Sight

The eye is probably the most highly developed of all the sense organs. The horse's eye is huge, one of the largest in the animal kingdom, larger than that of the whale and the elephant. It also possesses a light-intensifying modification known as the *tapetum lucidum*. This is a layer in the eye that reflects light back onto the retina, enabling horses to see in dim light. It can be seen to glow in the dark (similar to cats' eyes). This suggests that the horse evolved probably as a nocturnal animal, being most active at dawn and dusk.

The eyes are set high up on the head towards the side rather than at the front (Figure 10.5), giving the horse remarkable all round vision. The head is in turn set on a long, flexible neck. The eyes are set in bony sockets or orbits, which are positioned in the skull for maximum protection. The orbits contain large fat pads, which lie behind the eye and acts as a cushion.

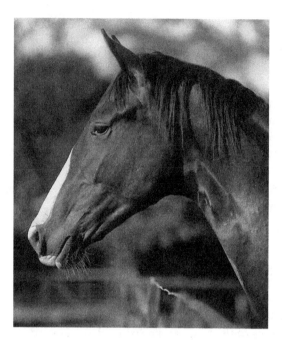

Figure 10.5 The eye is set high up towards the side of the head.

Unlike the spherical human eyeball, the horse's eyeball is slightly flattened from front to back, with the upper part being less flattened than the lower (Figure 10.6). This means that the retina is closer to the lens at the bottom of the eye than the top, so that both near and far objects can be seen at the same time, enabling horses to graze whilst keeping an eye on the horizon – a watch for potential danger.

Humans have an elastic lens and ciliary muscles, which help it to change shape and thereby focus on an object. The horse's lens is non-elastic, and the ciliary muscle is not as developed as that of humans. This means the horse does not use just the ciliary muscle to focus as humans do. Instead, the horse relies on moving its head up and down while the ciliary muscles move the lens back and forth slightly to bring the image to focus on the retina.

Since its eyes are located on each side of its head, the horse's vision is largely *monocular* (single-eyed), seeing its surroundings as two separate pictures, one from each eye. It has, however, some binocular vision directly in front of it. The horse has two blind spots: just in front before the range of the binocular vision and immediately behind his body (Figure 10.7). This is one reason why care should be taken when approaching horses from behind. The horse's muzzle also obscures its view, giving it only indistinct vision below eye level.

Like the human eye, it takes time for the eye to adapt when the horse moves from sun to shade.

Human

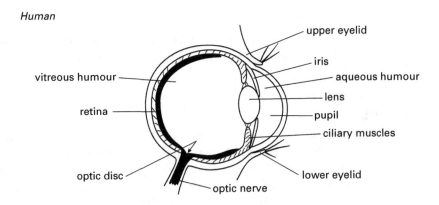

Horse

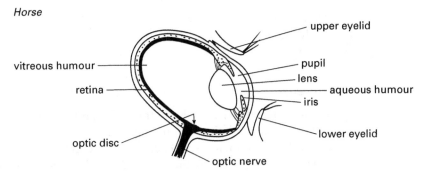

Figure 10.6 Comparison of the human and equine eye.

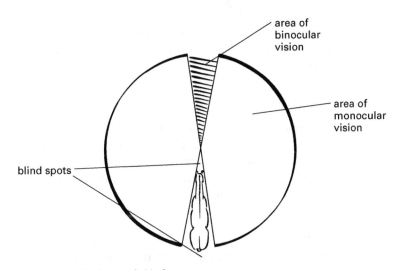

Figure 10.7 The horse's field of vision.

Colour vision

Horses are not colour blind. Horses have specialised colour-detecting cells known as *cones* in their retinas. They see yellow, orange and red best of all.

Hearing

Another sense, equally important to the horse, is that of hearing. Horses need their hearing to help them survive in the wild. They have a highly-developed and acute sense of hearing and their sensitive ears can detect a wide range of sounds from very low to very high frequencies. A horse can hear sounds that are outside of the human range.

The ear consists of three sections:

- Outer ear
- Middle ear
- Inner ear

Outer ear

The outer ear is the visible part of the ear, or *pinna*. The horse's excellent sense of hearing is helped by its highly mobile ears, which can move independently of each other. Each can rotate through 180° and is controlled by no fewer than 16 muscles, enabling the horse to pick up sounds from different directions without moving its whole body (Figure 10.8).

Horses also use their ears to give visual signals to other horses and humans. The position of the ears will give clues as to the horse's mood. Pricked ears are typical of horses that are alert, interested or startled. If the ears are pinned flat back, then this is a threat signal. In the wild, pinning back the ears was a protective measure in case of attack by a predator. If the ears are pinned back, they are less likely to be torn or damaged.

Middle ear

The middle ear is separated from the outer ear by the tympanic membrane, or eardrum, which is connected to three small bones with equestrian names, known (from outside in) as the *malleus* (hammer), *incus* (anvil) and *stapes* (stirrup). These little bones provide a mechanical link with the eardrum (Figure 10.9).

Inner ear

The inner ear is responsible for balance and informs the brain of the position of the horse's head at all times. It consists of a series of membranous

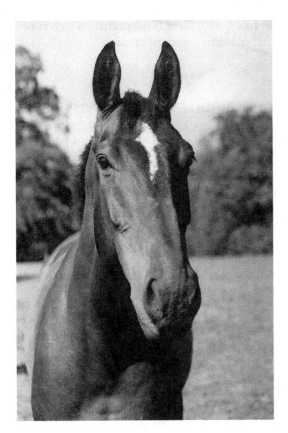

Figure 10.8 The horse has large mobile ears.

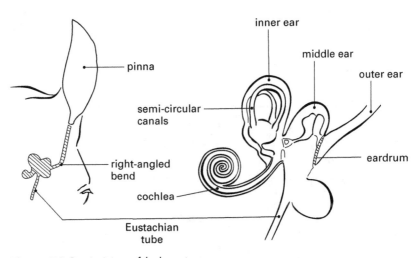

Figure 10.9 Anatomy of the horse's ear.

tubes (*labyrinth*), which are filled with fluid. This performs two functions, that of hearing and that of balance and orientation.

Guttural pouches

The horse is unique in that it has two large sacs connected to each of the two Eustachian tubes (one for each ear), known as the *guttural pouches*. They are situated between the pharynx and the skull and have a capacity of about 300 ml. The guttural pouches lie very close to important nerves and arteries and there is a condition known as Guttural Pouch Mycosis (caused by a fungus) which can be life threatening if the vital nerves and blood vessels become affected.

Taste and smell

The senses of taste and smell are very closely linked in horses, so much so that they are often thought to be inseparable.

Taste

Taste is an important factor in the ability of horses to select their food, particularly if they are deficient in some nutrient. Taste stimuli also increase stomach secretions.

Taste sensations are produced by minute raised areas on the tongue called *papillae*, on whose surface the taste buds are situated. The structure of a taste bud is shown in Figure 10.10. The highest concentration of taste cells is situated at the back of the tongue.

Although it is known that in man four specific tastes occur, i.e. sweet, salt, bitter and sour (acid), there are considerable differences between species. For example, it has been shown that whilst cats hate sugars

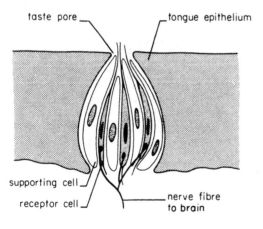

taste pore

tongue epithelium

supporting cell

receptor cell

nerve fibre
to brain

Figure 10.10   Structure of a taste bud.

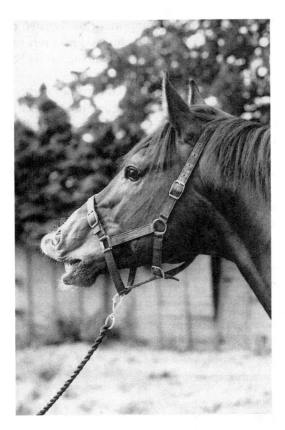

Figure 10.11 Flehmen.

and will avoid them, horses have shown a definite sweet tooth, hence their preference for sweet feed or molassed mixtures. It has also been shown that horses cannot distinguish between pure water and highly-concentrated sucrose (sugar) solutions, which are offensive to man. Taste can vary considerably though, within a species, so different horses will show individual preferences for different tastes. It is thought that this has a genetic base.

It has been proven in other animals, that if they are vitamin deficient, they will select foods high in that vitamin (if it is available to them). This ability to correct dietary deficiencies is lost if the sensory nerves to the taste buds are cut. Horses have a specific taste for salt, and will search it out if deficient. Therefore a salt lick should always be made available to them.

Smell

The sense of smell is important not only for seeking out and selecting food and water, but also as a communication system within groups of horses. The sense of smell is important for horses' reproductive patterns and social behaviour. Mares, for example, rely on their sense of smell to bond with their foals. As soon as the foal is born the mare will lick and smell the foal.

All horses have the ability to hold up their noses and curl the upper lip in a gesture known as Flehmen (Figure 10.11). This is often seen when horses are presented with a strange or strong smell, but it is most often seen in stallions in their courtship activity with mares that are in oestrus.

Horses also use this sense to smell droppings on the pasture or a patch of grass that has been staled upon by another horse. Stallions, or geldings showing stallion-like behaviour, will then dung on top of these smells to mark the territory as their own.

Summary points

- The nervous system has two parts, the CNS and PNS (including the autonomic nervous system)
- CNS consists of the brain and spinal cord
- PNS is made up mostly of communication nerves, which carry signals out of the CNS
- Nervous system responds to internal and external stimuli by initiating responses
- Links to all other body systems
- Much faster than the endocrine system
- Includes the sense organs

The Endocrine System

The word *hormone* is derived from the Greek *hormon* which means 'to arouse activity or stir up'. The endocrine system is composed of ductless glands that produce and secrete hormones, or chemical messengers, directly into the bloodstream to specific organs in the horse's body. These hormones act by controlling and affecting many body functions and organs, and are responsible for the horse's behaviour patterns.

Although the functions of the endocrine system are linked to those of the nervous system, it is much slower, but, because hormones are chemicals that are carried in the blood, they are longer-lasting than the quick, short-acting, electrical impulses carried by nerves. The positions of some of the horse's endocrine glands are shown in Figure 11.1.

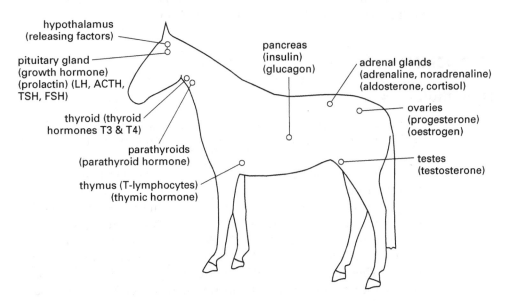

Figure 11.1 Position of the endocrine glands.

The most important endocrine glands are:

- Ovaries
- Testes
- Adrenal glands
- Pancreas
- Pituitary gland
- Hypothalamus
- Pineal gland
- Thyroid
- Parathyroids
- Thymus

Hormones are responsible for numerous body processes including:

- Puberty
- Growth
- Pregnancy and birth
- Lactation
- Aggression
- Metabolism
- Sexual development and function

All endocrine glands have a good blood supply, with capillaries running straight through them, so that when the hormones are manufactured they can be released immediately into the blood, without the need for ducts. Each gland produces specific hormones, and each hormone affects specific target organs.

ENDOCRINE GLANDS

Hypothalamus

Although the hypothalamus is not, strictly speaking, itself an endocrine gland, it does have indirect control over many of the endocrine glands via its effects on the pituitary gland. It is primarily concerned with hunger, thirst and other autonomic functions (see Chapter 10, p. 122).

Hormonal secretions by the various endocrine glands are under the control of the hypothalamus, which achieves this control by a negative feedback mechanism (Figure 11.2). When hormone levels become too high, they inhibit secretions by both the hypothalamus and pituitary glands. These glands respond by producing less stimulating hormone, thus reducing production by endocrine glands elsewhere in the body, so that blood levels of that hormone decline.

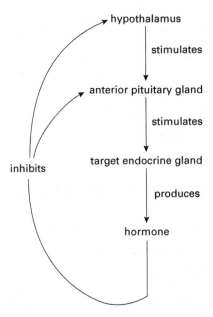

Figure 11.2 Negative feedback.

Pituitary

The pituitary gland is sometimes referred to as the master gland as it is generally accepted to be the single most important endocrine gland. It regulates and controls the activities of other endocrine glands and therefore many of the important body processes of the horse.

The pituitary gland is about the size of a pea and hangs down from the base of the brain where a stalk of nerve fibres attaches it to the hypothalamus. The pituitary gland consists of two lobes, known as the *anterior* and *posterior* lobes. These different lobes produce a range of hormones (Tables 11.1 and 11.2).

Thyroid gland

The thyroid gland consists of two lobes, one on each side of the windpipe at the level of the larynx, or voice box. It stimulates tissue metabolism, maintains the horse's basal metabolic rate and, through calcitonin synthesis, helps maintain the correct calcium and phosphorus balance. The thyroid produces the following hormones:

- *Thyroxin*
- *Triiodothyronine*
- *Calcitonin*

Thyroxine and triiodothyronine production are dependent upon iodine. A shortage of iodine will therefore affect these hormones.

Table 11.1   Hormones produced by the anterior lobe of the pituitary gland.

Hormone	Function
Growth hormone (GH)	Regulates height and growth; the main controller of the horse's final height
Thyrotrophin or thyroid stimulating hormone (TSH)	Controls the horse's thyroid gland
Adrenocorticotrophin (ACTH)	Controls adrenal cortex
Prolactin or lactogenic hormone (LTH)	Controls milk production during lactation
Gonadotrophins	Control sexual development and sex organs (ovaries and testes)
Follicle stimulating hormone (FSH)	Stimulates ovaries to produce *oestrogen* and ovulation in mares Stimulates sperm production in colts and stallions
Luteinising hormone (LH)	Stimulates ovaries to produce a *corpus luteum* from the ruptured follicle after ovulation, and to produce *progesterone*
Interstitial cell stimulating hormone (ICSH)	Stimulates sperm and testosterone production

Table 11.2   Hormones produced by the posterior lobe of the pituitary gland.

Hormone	Function
Antidiuretic hormone (ADH) or vasopressin	Regulates water absorption in the kidneys
Oxytocin	Contracts mammary glands to release milk to the foal when suckling Contracts uterine muscles to expel the foal during birth

Parathyroids

The parathyroid glands are a group of four small glands that lie behind the lobes of the thyroid gland in the horse's neck. They secrete parathyroid hormone (PTH), which helps to control blood calcium levels.

If blood calcium levels drop, PTH is released into the bloodstream. This causes the bones to release more calcium into the blood, the gut to absorb more calcium from food and the kidneys to conserve calcium. These effects quickly restore the blood calcium level. If blood calcium levels rise, the amount of PTH secretion is reduced and the above effects are reversed, with the horse's body storing more calcium in bone and excreting more calcium in the urine.

Adrenal glands

The adrenal glands lie next to and immediately above the kidneys. Each adrenal gland is divided into two distinct regions, the adrenal cortex, which forms the outer shell, and the adrenal medulla, which forms the centre of the gland.

Adrenal cortex

The adrenal cortex produces steroid hormones including:

- *Aldosterone* – regulates salts in the body, particularly sodium chloride (see Chapter 5, p. 61)
- *Cortisol* and *cortisone* – metabolise carbohydrates, fats and proteins; cortisol also helps to control inflammation and reduce the effects of shock
- *Sex hormones* – oestrogen and some progesterone in females, testosterone in the male

Adrenal medulla

The adrenal medulla produces *adrenaline* and *noradrenaline*. Often known as the stress hormones, they are produced in response to stress and increase the heart rate and blood pressure, slow down the digestive tract and urinary systems and increase blood sugar. All these are preparing the horse's body for fight or flight.

Pancreas

The pancreas is an elongated triangular-shaped gland that is situated behind the horse's stomach in a loop of small intestine.

Specialised areas throughout the pancreas form the endocrine part of the pancreas. This area consists of the Islets of Langerhans that secrete the hormones *glucagon* and *insulin*. Both insulin and glucagon are responsible for maintaining the blood glucose level within a normal range and diverting glucose to and from tissues.

Thymus

The thymus is situated just behind the sternum, between the horse's lungs. It is made up of two lobes joined together in front of the windpipe and below the level of the thyroid gland.

The thymus plays a role in the immune system by producing *thymosins*, which stimulate the development of *T-lymphocytes*. These are cells that are important in making antibodies to fight disease, and may also be instrumental in preventing cancer. The thymus is particularly active in foals. It is unusual in that it is active until puberty and then starts to lay down fat and become relatively inactive. The thymus produces lymphocytes, which are vital for the horse's defence system in its fight against disease.

Ovaries

As well as producing eggs, the ovaries are glands situated either side of the uterus that produce the female hormones *progesterone* and *oestrogen*. The oestrogens are responsible for the behavioural changes in the mare during her oestrus cycle. Progesterone has a role in the oestrus cycle and is also responsible for maintaining pregnancy in the early days after conception.

Testes

The testes are responsible for producing the male hormone testosterone, which produces the physical characteristics of the male horse. Testosterone is responsible for the increased musculature of stallions because it has an anabolic effect.

Pineal gland

This is a tiny structure located within the brain itself. It is responsible for secretion of the hormone *melatonin*. The amount of hormone secreted varies depending upon the day length, with more being produced during darkness, so that the blood levels of melatonin varies with the season. This has an effect on the mare's oestrus cycle, initiating oestrous activity as day length increases in the spring.

These annual cycles are called *circannual*, while the 24-hour cycles are called *circadian*. Behaviour that is based on these cycles are said to follow circannual/circadian *rhythms*.

Summary points

- Composed of ductless glands
- Produces chemical messengers or hormones
- Controls many body functions and behaviour
- Slower than the nervous system, but works with it
- Important for growth, metabolism, stress, kidney function, digestive system and the reproductive cycle

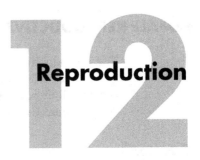

Reproduction

The survival of any species is dependent upon the reproductive success of the generations that follow each other. Genetic material, in the form of genes, is passed from one generation to another at the time of conception (Figure 12.1).

The organs that enable horses to reproduce make up the reproductive system, which has three functions:

- Production of the sex cells or gametes – male sperm and female eggs
- Brings egg and sperm together at mating for fertilisation
- Nourishes and protects the resulting embryo

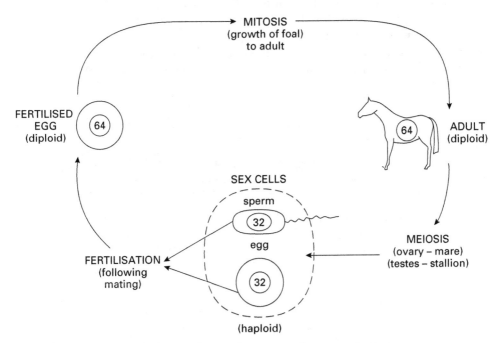

Figure 12.1 Life cycle of the horse, showing the positions of mitosis and meiosis.

FEMALE REPRODUCTIVE ANATOMY

The reproductive system of the mare consists of two *ovaries* and the *genital tract*, which is composed of the *Fallopian tubes, uterus, cervix* and *vagina*. All these are suspended within the body cavity from a sheet of strong connective tissue known as the *broad ligament* (Figure 12.2).

Ovaries

The ovaries are situated between the last rib and the point of hip, and they contain the mare's eggs, or *ova*. The ovaries are also responsible for the production of the female hormone *oestrogen*. Each mare is born with several hundred thousand immature eggs and no more will be produced during her lifetime.

There is little ovarian activity until puberty, which, in the mare, takes place between her first and second years. Fillies are often seen in oestrus during the yearling spring/summer, but under natural conditions it is unusual for fillies to foal until they are over three years old.

Following puberty, and under hormonal control, eggs mature and one is released from the ovaries at regular intervals during each oestrus cycle. Each egg begins as a primordial germ cell, surrounded by a gradually-enlarging fluid-filled sac known as a *Graafian follicle* (Figure 12.3). At oestrus this mature follicle breaks open, or *ruptures*, and the egg is released into the widened end of the *Fallopian tube* in a process known as *ovulation*.

The ruptured follicle then becomes a structure known as the *corpus luteum*, or 'yellow body', which begins to secrete the hormone

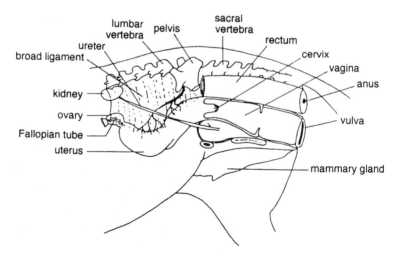

Figure 12.2 Reproductive tract of the mare.

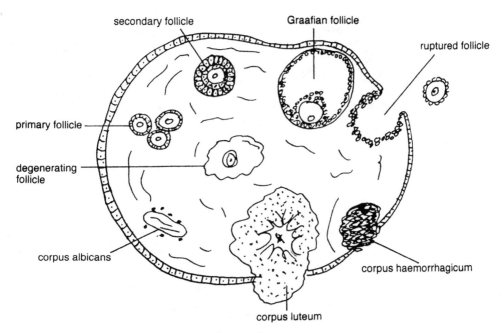

secondary follicle   Graafian follicle

ruptured follicle

primary follicle

degenerating follicle

corpus albicans

corpus haemorrhagicum

corpus luteum

Figure 12.3   Section through an ovary of a sexually active mare.

progesterone. If a pregnancy is not established, the corpus luteum will eventually become non-functional, its cells being replaced by scar tissue.

Fallopian tubes

Also known as *oviducts,* these tubes carry the ovulated mature egg to the uterine horn. The Fallopian tubes are coiled and are approximately 20–30 cm long, and 2–3 mm in diameter. The ovarian end of the Fallopian tube is funnel shaped. Sperm, if present, will fertilise the egg in the Fallopian tube before the resulting embryo passes into the uterus. Only fertilised eggs will pass into the uterus. Normally the non-fertilised eggs will remain in the Fallopian tubes where they eventually disintegrate.

Uterus

The uterus of the horse is a muscular sac, which consists of two horns, a body and a neck (*cervix*) (Figure 12.4). In horses, the embryo will develop in the horn of the uterus, whereas in humans the embryo develops in its body.

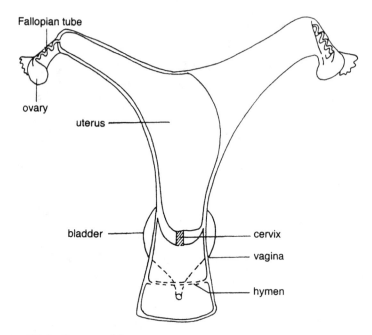

Figure 12.4 Structure of the uterus.

Cervix

The uterus is separated from the vagina by a neck, or cervix. This is a constricted part of the uterus and is usually about 7 cm long and 4 cm in diameter.

The cervix plays a vital role in protecting both the foetus and the mare by being tightly closed when the mare is pregnant or not in season, preventing the entrance of infection to the womb. The cervix is capable of rapid dilation just prior to birth.

Vagina

The vagina consists of a muscular tube, which is approximately 20 cm long and 12 cm in diameter and extends from the cervix to the vulva.

Vulva

This is the external opening of the mare's genital tract. The lips of the vulva are arranged vertically on either side of the vulval opening and are situated immediately below the anus. They are normally held fairly tightly together to form the *vulval seal* (Figure 12.5).

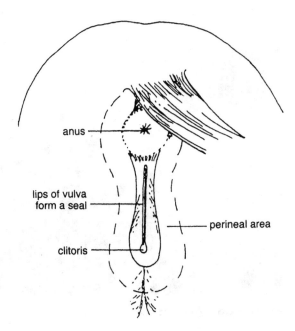

Figure 12.5 Vulval seal.

OESTROUS CYCLE

Oestrus cycle is the term used to describe the alternating periods of sexual activity in the mare. It is controlled by hormones, which are initially secreted by the pituitary gland.

Mares begin having oestrus cycles at puberty, which is usually around one and a half years of age. The cycle has two phases, that of *oestrus* ('heat'; 'in season'), when the mare is receptive to the stallion and ovulation takes place, and that of *dioestrus* (between oestrus periods), when the mare is not receptive. The cycle typically lasts 21 days in the mare, oestrus lasting for approximately five days and dioestrus for 15–16 days. Ovulation usually occurs on the last but one or last day of the oestrus period, and this is fairly constant no matter what the length of oestrus is.

The mare is said to be *seasonally anoestrous*, which means that she will only display oestrous activity for six months of the year, typically April to September. This means that the resulting foals will be born 11 months later, in March to August, when food will be plentiful and the environmental temperature not too low, increasing the foal's chances of survival.

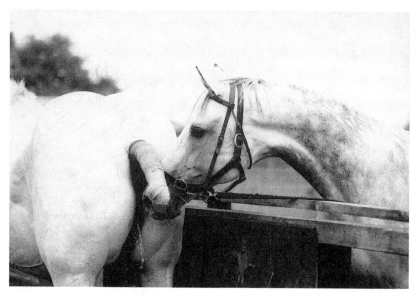

Figure 12.6 Mare in season.

Behavioural signs of oestrus

As oestrus approaches, mares will often become restless and irritable. A urinating posture is adopted whilst repeatedly exposing or 'winking' the clitoris (Figure 12.6). The stallion will often exhibit Flehmen, with the upper lip rolled up and the neck stretched outwards and upwards (Figure 10.11), when the mare is in season. This is in response to pheromones present in the mare's urine.

Hormonal changes during the oestrus cycle

The physical and behavioural changes that occur in mares throughout each cycle are controlled by chemical messenger substances called hormones (see Chapter 11, pp. 133–8). The hormonal changes associated with oestrus are summarised in Figures 12.7 and 12.8 and are as follows:

- Environmental factors, such as increasing day length, nutrition and warmth, stimulate the hypothalamus to secrete the hormone *gonadotrophin releasing hormone* (GnRH), which in turn begins the onset of oestrous activity in spring.
- GnRH causes the release by the pituitary gland, of *follicle stimulating hormone* (FSH), which causes the follicles to develop within the ovary. As these follicles grow they secrete oestrogen. These hormones are responsible for the changes in the mare's behaviour and physical changes in the genital tract.

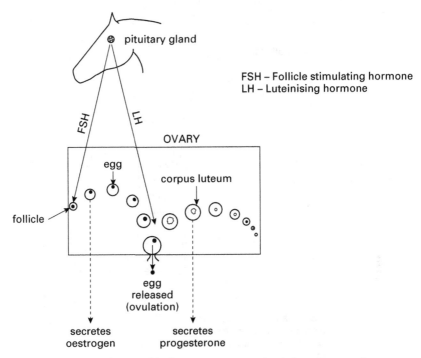

Figure 12.7 Production of the hormones associated with the oestrous cycle.

- Rising levels of oestrogen then stimulate the pituitary gland to produce *luteinising hormone* (LH) and to reduce the amount of FSH being secreted. Ovulation occurs under the influence of LH and the egg is released into the Fallopian tube ready for possible fertilisation. The *corpus luteum* (yellow body) is then formed in place of the burst follicle within the ovary, and this produces the hormone *progesterone*. This hormone has an effect opposite to that of oestrogen. Progesterone prepares the uterus to receive a fertilised egg and is essential for maintaining pregnancy.
- Once ovulation has occurred and the follicle has burst, oestrogen production from the follicle declines. This, combined with the rise in progesterone from the *corpus luteum*, is responsible for the changes in behaviour and genital tract of the mare that occur after ovulation. The mare then goes out of season (generally 24 hours post ovulation).
- If fertilisation takes place, then the *corpus luteum* continues to produce progesterone to maintain the pregnancy. If fertilisation does not occur, the uterus produces a substance known as *prostaglandin* (PGF$_{2\alpha}$), which effectively kills off the *corpus luteum* in the ovary. As a result, progesterone secretion falls and this causes the anterior pituitary to secrete FSH and the cycle starts all over again.

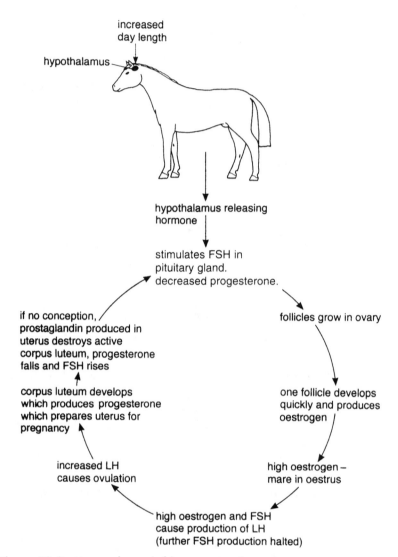

Figure 12.8 Hormonal control of the oestrous cycle.

Foal heat

After foaling, the mare should return to oestrus in 5–10 days. This is known as the *foal heat*, and usually lasts for only 2–4 days.

MALE REPRODUCTIVE ANATOMY

The male reproductive organs consist of the *testes* (testicles) which are held within the *scrotum*, the *epididymis*, *vas deferens*, the *accessory glands* and the *penis* (Figure 12.9).

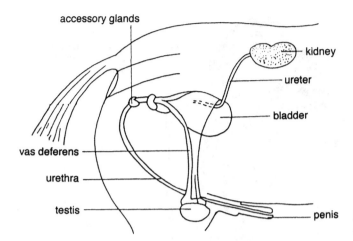

Figure 12.9 Reproductive anatomy of the stallion.

Scrotum

The testes are carried in a sac known as the *scrotum*, which is situated between the hind legs of the stallion. It is outside of the body because the temperature inside the body is too high for sperm development, while the temperature within the scrotum is approximately 4–7°C cooler than within the body itself. The scrotum is designed to lose heat when the external temperature is warm. When it is cold, a muscle known as the cremaster muscle pulls the testis against the body to reduce heat loss.

Testes

The stallion normally has two testes. They are egg-shaped, and each mature testis measures approximately 6–12 cm long, 5 cm wide and 4–7 cm high.

In the foetus, the testes develop near the kidneys, well inside the horse's body cavity. Approximately one month before birth, the testes begin their descent into the scrotum, although they are very small at this stage. Newborn foals normally have both testes in the scrotum at birth or soon after. By the time the horse is two years old, the testes have reached their full size. Their growth is controlled by hormones that also control sperm production.

Once the testes are mature, the male hormone *testosterone* is produced. Each testis consists of a mass of tiny tubes known as the *seminiferous tubules*. Within these small tubules are the cells that divide to form the sperm. These cells also produce testosterone. The seminiferous

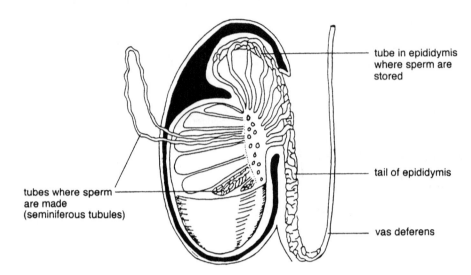

Figure 12.10 Section through a testis.

tubules all join up and converge towards the front of the testis where they pass into a structure known as the *epididymis* (Figure 12.10).

The whole cycle of sperm development within the testes takes 50–60 days in the stallion. The mean daily production of sperm is in the order of 7×10^9. The more a stallion is used, i.e. the higher the frequency of ejaculation, the faster the sperm are produced.

Semen, otherwise known as the *ejaculate* is made up of both sperm and seminal fluid (produced by the accessory sex glands).

Epididymis

The epididymis is a U-shaped, coiled tube, which collects the sperm produced by the seminiferous tubules and connects with the *vas deferens*. Sperm are immature when they leave the testis and must undergo a maturation period before they are capable of fertilisation. The epididymis serves as a holding area in which sperm can mature prior to ejaculation.

Vas deferens

The vas deferens is a muscular tube, which, at the time of ejaculation, propels the sperm and associated fluids from the epididymis to the *urethra* (the tube which carries urine from the bladder to the end of the penis).

Accessory sex glands

During ejaculation, these glands secrete 60–90% of the total volume of the ejaculate. These glands supply a favourable medium for the carriage and nourishment of mature sperm. The accessory glands consist of the *vesicular* gland (seminal vesicles), the *prostate* and the *bulbourethral* (Cowper's) glands.

Penis

The penis is the male organ of copulation and has three parts:

- *Glans* (free extremity)
- *Body* (main portion)
- *Two roots* (attach penis to pelvis)

The internal structure of the penis consists of erectile (or *cavernous*) tissue. Erection occurs when the penis becomes engorged with blood when the stallion is sexually stimulated. More blood enters the penis through the arterial supply than leaves through the veins. This increased blood volume, makes the penis bigger. On erection the penis of the horse doubles in length and thickness. A prominent margin or rose surrounds the end of the glans penis. This enlarges to three times its resting size after ejaculation. The end of the urethra projects through this rose.

PREGNANCY AND BIRTH

Fertilisation

This is the joining of an egg with a sperm, which takes place in the mare's Fallopian tube. Following mating, ejaculation by the stallion delivers millions of sperm into the uterus of the mare. These then swim towards the egg by whipping their tails, and eventually one will force itself through the outer jelly-like layer of the egg. To prevent several sperm penetrating the egg at the same time, an almost immediate block is set up after the first sperm has penetrated the inner membrane known as the vitelline membrane.

Once the sperm has penetrated the egg, it injects its own genes into it (Figure 12.11). Both egg and sperm have half the number of chromosomes of all the other cells of the horse's body, so that at fertilisation the foetus will have the full number of chromosomes required.

Egg (32) + Sperm (32) = Embryo (64)

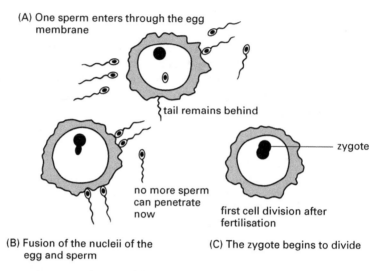

Figure 12.11   Fertilisation of the ovum.

Pregnancy (gestation)

In the few weeks immediately following fertilisation, the cells of the embryo start to multiply in number by the process of mitosis and develop, or *differentiate*, into different types of tissue – tissue for the future skeleton, muscles, organs, etc. Gradually the embryo grows into something that looks like a miniature horse. This is the *foetus*.

For the first three to four weeks of pregnancy, a *yolk sac* provides the embryo with nutrients. This yolk sac is quite large in horses compared with other animals. The foetus is free floating within the uterus at this time. At around day 38, cells of the foetus attach to the uterus lining, forming structures known as *endometrial cups*. These are unique to the horse family. The endometrial cups secrete a hormone called *pregnant mare serum gonadotrophin* (PMSG), which is essential for the maintenance of the pregnancy in the early days.

From days 40–150 of pregnancy, the *placenta* develops to full working order, attaching the foetus to the mare's uterus and providing it with a blood supply. The horse's placenta covers the entire uterine surface. There is a thin barrier separating the foetal blood circulation from the mare's, and this allows diffusion of substances between the mare and foetus. As blood flows through the placenta it picks up oxygen and soluble food from the mare's blood supply, at the same time passing urea and carbon dioxide back into the mare's blood supply. Antibodies also cross to the foetus via the placenta, helping to protect the newborn foal from disease after birth. Although the blood supplies are close to each other, they do not mix.

As the embryo develops in the mare's uterus, a membrane known as the *amnion* surrounds it. The amnion forms a fluid-filled sac around the embryo, protecting it. The fluid is called *amniotic fluid*. As the embryo increases in size, so does the amnion. The foetus floats in the middle of it.

The average length of pregnancy in mares is around eleven months, or 333–336 days from the date of conception and the highly-muscular uterus expands greatly during this time.

It is the foetus that determines the time of birth as the mare approaches the end of her pregnancy – otherwise known as being *full term*. Various factors are involved in this timing, including:

- Genetics
- Nutrition
- Environmental factors

Signs of imminent foaling

A mare will normally start to bag-up about three weeks before foaling. Her udder becomes progressively larger, until a waxy discharge of dried milk can be seen on the teats; this often indicates that the mare will foal in the next 24 hours, but it is possible for a mare to foal without waxing-up. Mares may also run milk prior to foaling and this can result in the loss of vital colostrum.

Signs of imminent foaling are:

- Waxing up
- Changes in behaviour (especially tending to stand away from other mares)
- Elongation of the vulva
- Relaxing of the pelvic muscles causing indentation of the croup

Once the mare has waxed up, foaling is imminent and she should not be left unattended for long periods of time. Mares are kept under close observation at this time and disturbance is kept to a minimum. Mares normally foal at night and do not appreciate outside interference.

Birth (parturition)

The birth of the foal marks the end of pregnancy; the foal is pushed through the birth canal by contractions of the uterus and abdominal muscles. At the start of birth the foal is usually lying on its back with its head, neck and legs flexed. As the contractions begin the foal extends its forelimbs and head, turning into an upright position with its forelegs and muzzle pressed against the cervix.

During the first stage of labour powerful contractions cause a rise in pressure in the fluids surrounding the foetus and these press against the placenta. As the cervix dilates it leaves a weak spot through which the placental membranes bulge until they rupture, releasing the allantoic fluid. This breaking of the waters marks the end of the first stage. The cervix is now fully dilated and the foal is pushed through the birth canal by contractions of the uterus and abdominal muscles.

Stages of foaling

There are three stages of foaling:

- The first stage is measured from the first contractions until the breaking of the waters; as in humans, this may be a very short time or several hours
- The second stage is from the breaking of the waters until the birth of the foal
- The third stage is from the actual birth of the foal until the expulsion of the afterbirth

First stage

During the first stage of labour, the foal turns from lying on its back (head to the rear end of the mare) to an upright position in which its forelegs and head are at the entrance of the pelvic canal.

Mares will show a range of signs, including:

- Looking at their flanks
- Sweating
- Showing Flehmen (curled top lip with head and neck outstretched)
- Pacing the box and pawing at the ground

Uterine contractions are starting during first stage labour, and they continue until the pressure created in the uterus is sufficient to rupture the allantois at the opening to the cervix. The resultant rush of allantoic fluid (breaking waters) indicates the start of second stage labour. This is often confused with the mare urinating.

Second stage

Second stage labour will normally last for about 25 minutes, but may last from ten minutes to one hour. It commences when the waters break and a rush of fluid appears as the allantois ruptures. The mare may be uncomfortable at this stage, and will sometimes lie down and stand up several times.

An opaque whitish-blue bag will appear (the amnion). This has a balloon-like appearance and should contain one of the foal's fore-feet. The foal should be presented in a diving position, and its second leg and head must be in the correct position for birth to proceed normally.

The most difficult stage of the birth process occurs when the foal's shoulders pass through the pelvis (this normally corresponds with the time when the foal's poll passes through the vulva). The second leg always follows the first in a way that will slant the foal's shoulders, enabling it to pass more easily out of the mare's pelvis.

After some less violent contractions by the mare, the foal is born, and at this stage the umbilical cord is intact. More often than not the cord will break naturally when either mare or foal moves. It is important that this happens gradually and naturally as, whilst the umbilical cord is intact, the foal will still be receiving valuable nutrients and oxygen from the mare.

Third stage

Third stage labour commences when the foal is born and the umbilical cord has ruptured, and it involves the expulsion of the placenta (or afterbirth). The mare will usually expel it within about half an hour.

Careful examination of the afterbirth is essential to ensure that it is complete – it is possible for the tip of the non-pregnant horn to tear, leaving a section of placenta remaining in the uterus. Placental retention can have a very serious effect causing widespread infection (toxaemia) and laminitis.

Colostrum

For the first month of its life, the foal is unable to manufacture significant levels of antibodies, and therefore has limited natural defences against infections or disease unless it acquires immunity from the mare. Some antibodies are not able to cross from the uterine blood to the placental blood, but are transmitted in the mare's first milk, which is known as *colostrum*.

Colostrum contains high levels of antibodies, which the gut can absorb for as few as only 12–48 hours, after which the foal will be able to manufacture its own. Failure to absorb sufficient antibodies from colostrum will leave the foal susceptible to disease, and this may happen if the mare runs a significant amount of milk before foaling or if the foal fails to suckle. In the latter case, the mare may have to be milked and the foal bottle fed until it has the strength to feed on its own.

Summary points

- Reproduction is vital for the survival of the equine species
- Mating results in the fusion of an egg and a sperm cell
- Reproductive organs are very different in the male and female, unlike any other organs of the body
- Oestrous cycle of the mare is typically 21 days
- Oestrous cycle is under hormonal control
- Sperm development takes approximately 50–60 days in the stallion
- There are three separate stages of foaling

Disease-causing Organisms

The horse is continually challenged by disease-causing organisms of one sort or another. These organisms are often referred to as 'germs', but may be broadly categorised into one of two groups: micro-organisms and parasites. Disease-causing micro-organisms may cause harm by:

- Attacking and destroying cells within the horse's body
- Releasing poisonous substances, known as toxins, which enter the bloodstream

Parasites may live within the horse's body or on the surface. These include the single-celled parasites known as *protoctista* (*protozoa*), worms, mites and insects. Colonisation by parasites (worms, mites and insects) tends to be referred to as an infestation rather than as an infection.

Some micro-organisms are *pathogenic* (cause disease), whereas others are required and helpful to the horse. An example of this is the millions of micro-organisms present in the horse's gut (see Chapter 4, p. 51). In fact, without them the horse could not digest its herbage diet. Another example would be the millions of bacteria which live naturally on the horse's skin without producing any signs of disease.

Organisms which cause disease are known as *pathogens*. Most diseases that affect horses are caused by the micro-organisms *bacteria* and *viruses*. Horses may be susceptible to some micro-organisms but not to others. This is because many micro-organisms are species specific. For example, horses cannot catch influenza from humans.

In the middle of the nineteenth century, a scientist known as Louis Pasteur showed that microbes that spoil food came from the surrounding air. Further work by scientists showed that diseases were caused by specific bacteria.

Micro-organisms vary in their ability to invade and multiply, a capacity known as virulence. Sometimes they may spread from a part of the horse's body where they are normally harmless to another part

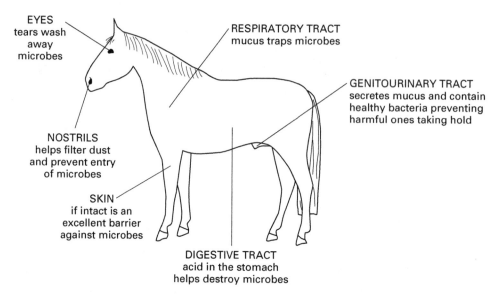

EYES
tears wash
away
microbes

RESPIRATORY TRACT
mucus traps microbes

GENITOURINARY TRACT
secretes mucus and contain
healthy bacteria preventing
harmful ones taking hold

NOSTRILS
helps filter dust
and prevent entry
of microbes

SKIN
if intact is an
excellent barrier
against microbes

DIGESTIVE TRACT
acid in the stomach
helps destroy microbes

Figure 13.1   Possible entrance sites for micro-organisms.

where they become harmful. An example of this is when there is leakage from the horse's gut into the surrounding abdominal space. This results in infection of the gut lining or *peritoneum*, which is known as *peritonitis*. The entry of micro-organisms from the soil into wounds or during surgery can also introduce localised infection, which may become systemic.

Horses suffering from disease will commonly show signs of illness and these are known as *signs* or *symptoms*. Infection may take place through one of several routes (Figure 13.1). These possible entrance sites for micro-organisms include the eyes, mouth, nostrils, skin and the genitals. All these areas have mechanisms to reduce the possibility of pathogenic micro-organisms taking hold.

Should they get past the horse's protective mechanisms, infections normally produce a response from the horse's immune system, which attempts to fight the disease. In some cases, infection does spread throughout the horse's body, though, and this is termed a *systemic infection*. Infection may also be localised within a particular area or tissue.

Once inside the body, these organisms multiply rapidly. This stage of infection is known as the incubation period. Several weeks may go by before the horse shows symptoms of illness. A high temperature is often a feature of many infections in horses. Apart from diseases in which the symptoms and signs are easily recognisable, such as tetanus or strangles, diagnosis will often rely upon the isolation of the causative micro-organism.

Spread of disease

Disease may be spread from one horse to another, as with equine influenza, or it may be contracted from the environment. When large numbers of horses are affected it is known as an *epidemic*; if it is a worldwide infection, it becomes a *pandemic*.

Diseases are spread because micro-organisms get passed from one horse to another. Such diseases are termed *infectious*.

During the incubation period, just after infection when the pathogen is multiplying, horses will have micro-organisms within the body without showing any external signs of disease. These horses are termed *carriers*. Carriers may be infectious without showing symptoms of the disease.

Disease may be spread in several ways, including:

- Droplets in the air
- Dust
- Direct contact, touch
- Food or water supply
- Animal carriers (*vectors*), such as insects
- Body fluids, e.g. transmissible sexual diseases

MICRO-ORGANISMS

Bacteria

Bacteria are very small, living, single-celled micro-organisms, and they may be found almost anywhere – in air, water and soil. Some are useful, but many cause disease. Their structure is simpler than that of other organisms – for example, they do not contain a proper nucleus (Figure 13.2).

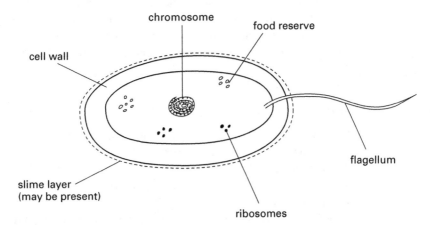

Figure 13.2   Basic structure of a bacterium.

Table 13.1   Some infectious diseases caused by bacteria.

Disease	Causative bacterium
Tetanus	Clostridium tetani
Strangles	Streptococcus equi
Botulism	Clostridium botulinum

Many bacteria are capable of surviving extreme conditions, such as drought, heat and cold, and have different ways of achieving this. Some bacteria can produce protective coats inside which they become dormant. When external conditions become beneficial, the bacteria 'wake' and become active again. Some bacteria may remain dormant for up to 50 years. *Spore-producing* bacteria include the *clostridial* organisms responsible for tetanus and botulism. These spores are able to lie dormant within the soil for many years. When a horse has a wound (often very minor) the tetanus-causing bacteria (*Clostridium tetani*) can enter the body via this route.

Pathogenic bacteria can be classified on the basis of their shape, into three main groups:

(1) *Cocci* (spherical)
(2) *Bacilli* (rod-shaped)
(3) *Spirochaetes* or *spirilla* (spiral)

Diseases caused by the cocci include pneumonia and strangles. Tetanus and botulism are caused by bacilli (Table 13.1).

Many bacteria that invade the horse's body thrive in warm, moist conditions. Some bacteria are *aerobic* which means that they require oxygen to grow and survive. They are therefore found in such places as the respiratory system or on the skin. *Anaerobic* bacteria, on the other hand, thrive in areas low in oxygen, such as deep in wounds or tissues.

Many bacteria are naturally static and only move around the horse's body in currents of fluid or air. Others are mobile and have filamentous tails to help them move.

Antibiotics

The horse's body will attempt to fight invading bacteria, and sometimes this is enough and the horse will recover without treatment (see Immune system, this chapter, p. 162). In many cases, though, treatment will be necessary, usually given as antibiotics either orally, in the feed, or by injection.

Some antibiotics such as penicillin are *bactericidal*, which means they kill invading bacteria. Others, such as tetracycline, are *bacteriostatic*

– they stop the bacteria from multiplying, enabling the body's own immune defences to overcome them.

Some micro-organisms are able to produce substances which defend them against the action of other micro-organisms. An example of this is the fungus penicillium which produces a substance which acts against bacteria. The substance was isolated by a famous scientist, Alexander Fleming, in 1928 and the substance is known as *penicillin*.

Penicillin is one of a range of drugs known as antibiotics which are used today to help treat diseases of horses. Although antibiotics are highly successful against bacteria, they do not have any effect on viruses. In addition, new strains of bacteria evolve which are resistant to antibiotics.

Viruses

Viruses are much smaller than bacteria. They are not even cells. A virus is approximately one hundredth the size of a bacterium and is approximately ten thousandth of a millimetre wide. Viruses have a much simpler structure than bacteria (Figure 13.3). They consist of a coiled thread of genetic material surrounded by a protein wall and are able to reproduce themselves only within living cells of the host animal in a process known as *replication* (see p. 160).

Despite their minute size, viruses can be extremely harmful. Many diseases in horses, including equine influenza, are caused by viruses. Viral infections vary from relatively minor problems, such as warts, to extremely serious diseases such as rabies. It is thought that some viral infections also lead to cancer. Viruses are grouped into families, some of which are shown in Table 13.2.

Viruses can enter the horse's body through all possible entrance routes: they may be inhaled in droplets or swallowed in food or water; they may be passed into the body through the saliva of biting insects, as is the case with equine infectious anaemia; they may enter the horse's body during covering.

Fighting viral infections is very difficult because it is almost impossible to design drugs which will 'kill' viruses without affecting the host

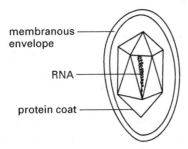

Figure 13.3 Basic structure of a virus.

Table 13.2   Common virus families.

Family	Diseases caused
Papovaviruses	Warts
Adenoviruses	Respiratory and eye infections Colds
Herpes viruses	Equine herpes virus 1 (EHV-1) and subtypes 1 (abortion strain) and 2 (respiratory strain) EHV-3 – coital exanthema
Orthomyxoviruses	Equine influenza

cell that the virus has colonised. Some antiviral agents, which prevent viruses from entering the host cells in the first place, or interfere with viral replication, have been produced in human medicine.

Immunisation can be a much more effective method of eradicating or reducing the effects of viruses. Vaccination programmes are used widely for the control of equine diseases such as equine influenza.

Replication

Technically, viruses do not reproduce themselves. Instead, they undergo a process known as *replication* (Figure 13.4). The virus invades the host cell and begins the process of making copies of itself from materials within the host cell itself – it is as though the host cell were a factory whose reproduction systems have been taken over. Thousands of new viruses may be released from one cell and these then attack new host cells. Different viruses attack different groups of cells, for example the equine influenza virus attacks cells of the respiratory tract. Not all viruses replicate as soon as they enter the horse's body, some just stay and wait, sometimes for years.

Defence against micro-organisms

Disinfection and sterilisation

Probably the most effective method of keeping micro-organisms out of the horse's body is to remove them from the environment. High-temperature treatment at 120°C for 15 minutes is enough to kill most germs. This process is known as *sterilisation*. An autoclave is used for this purpose, and veterinary surgeons use one to sterilise surgical instruments prior to surgery.

Places that need cleaning of germs, such as stables that have housed infected horses or loose boxes used at race courses for many different

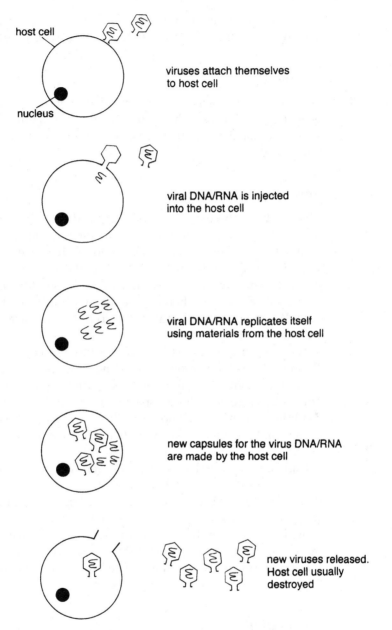

Figure 13.4 Viral replication.

horses, may be cleaned with disinfectant. Disinfectant is used routinely in studs and training stables to reduce the risk of disease.

Quarantine

Horses that have a serious infectious disease or that are known carriers of an infectious disease should be kept apart from others. These horses should be isolated until they are no longer infectious. This is known as quarantine.

Immune system

When a horse becomes infected with a disease, substances known as *antigens* on the surface of the micro-organism cause specialised white blood cells in the horse's body to produce chemicals known as *antibodies*. These antibodies then destroy the antigens. Following this chain of events, *memory cells* remain in the horse's blood, ready to produce antibodies again should the antigen infect the body for a second time. When horses make antibodies to fight a disease it is known as *active immunity*.

Tetanus, for example, is a serious bacterial disease affecting horses. Tetanus affects the nervous system and causes extremely painful and often lethal symptoms if it remains untreated. Muscles all over the horse's body go into painful spasm, including the horse's jaw, so this condition is commonly known as 'lockjaw'. The germs are found in the soil and are often picked up when the horse cuts itself or pricks its hoof.

If an infected horse has not already been vaccinated, it is too late for a vaccine to have any effect. The vet will therefore administer antibodies that have already been made in another horse, injecting the ill horse with tetanus antiserum. This is a useful treatment in an emergency as it provides instant antibodies. This is known as *passive immunity*. The instant antibodies are gradually broken down by the horse's body. For long-term protection, horses need to make their own antibodies (active immunity) and this is achieved by vaccination.

Vaccination

Vaccination provides protection against disease. It is a procedure by which the horse's own immune system is stimulated by injecting killed or weakened micro-organisms, or parts of them, into the horse. These weakened organisms are not able to cause disease. These micro-organisms then sensitise the immune system so that if the same micro-organism is encountered at a later date, it will quickly be dealt with by the action of the antibodies which have now been primed to act. The antibodies may either kill the germ itself or neutralise the toxin it produces.

Vaccines are now available to protect the horse against a wide range of infectious diseases, including influenza, rhinopneumonitis (EHV-1), eastern and western encephalomyelitis, rabies and strangles.

Different vaccines have varying durations of effectiveness. Boosters are often required at regular intervals to maintain the immune status. Equine influenza virus is able to mutate or change the shape of its outer coat. Vaccine manufacturers therefore have to continually update vaccines to cope with different strains of the equine influenza virus.

FUNGI

Fungi are much larger than bacteria and viruses, but they are relatively simple parasites. There are more than 100,000 species of fungus, and the group includes moulds, mildews, yeasts, mushrooms and toadstools. Most of these are harmless, and may even be beneficial. Some moulds, for example, are used to make antibiotics.

Some fungi, such as the yeasts, occur as colonies of individual cells. Others form chains of tubes or filaments called *hyphae*, which are formed into a complex network known as a *mycelium*. Many fungi form millions of tiny spores which can be carried in the air and remain dormant until suitable conditions are available for them to grow. Fungal spores are found mainly in the soil. They can penetrate into the tissues of the horse, as is the case with aspergillus, which causes infection of the mucous membranes and guttural pouch. Some fungal spores, particularly those found in mouldy hay, can cause damage when inhaled by horses, causing persistent allergic reactions in the lungs or COPD. The principal culprits here are *Micropolyspora faeni* and *Aspergillus fumigatus*.

Some yeasts are present normally within the horse's gut, where they may become a problem if the gut flora that normally keeps them under control are upset or disrupted by the use of antibiotics. They can then overgrow the bacterial population because antibiotics have no effect on fungi.

Probably the most common fungal infection of the horse is ringworm. Both *Trichophyton* and *Microsporum* species cause ringworm. In addition, fungi can cause disease in other ways. Certain fungi that infect food crops, for instance, produce dangerous toxins.

Antifungal drugs can be used to treat ringworm. These work by damaging the cell walls of the fungi, causing eventual death of the fungal cells.

PARASITES

Both internal and external parasites infect the horse. The most common internal parasites of horses are worms. External parasites include lice, ticks, mites and several species of flies.

Internal parasites (worms)

Worms that live within the horse's body tissues are true parasites in that they use the horse as a source of nutrition and a protected environment. All horses carry parasitic worm infections, and it has been estimated that a horse may pass as many as ten million worm eggs in their dung daily.

Once these eggs have passed onto the pasture, they may then develop into *larvae* (an immature form of the adult worm) that, at some time in their development, become infective to the horse. These infective larvae are taken into the horse's body as it grazes and then, depending upon the species, the larvae migrate through body tissues such as blood vessels, liver, lungs and the gut lining (*peritoneum*) before returning to the gut as adult worms. Here they lay eggs, so completing their life cycle. The life cycle of the large redworm (*Strongylus vulgaris*) is shown in Figure 13.5.

Worm infestations can pose quite severe health threats to horses, particularly when there are large numbers of immature larvae migrating

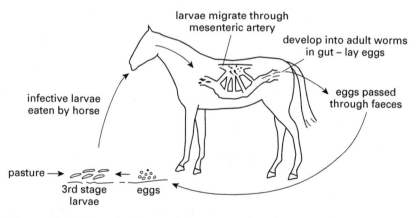

Figure 13.5 Life cycle of large redworm (*Strongylus vulgaris*).

Table 13.3 The major parasitic worms affecting horses.

Worm	Migratory behaviour	Adult behaviour
Large strongyles – Strongylus vulgaris; Strongylus edentatus	S. vulgaris migrates through blood vessels; damage may occur to blood vessels supplying the gut	Suck on plugs of bowel, causing localised bleeding; may interfere with digestion
Small strongyles – Trichonema; small redworm	Enter gut wall; may remain dormant for up to two years within sealed nodules; may interfere with nutrient absorption; release of large numbers simultaneously may lead to diarrhoea	Interfere with digestion of nutrients
Ascarids (roundworm)	Damage to lungs as larvae migrate through them; coughing, nasal discharge	Bowel obstruction and interference with digestion
Oxyuris (pinworm)	No migratory stage	Interfere with digestion; eggs deposited around anus cause irritation
Gasterophilus (bot)	Eggs laid on hairs of forelegs and chest; larvae migrate through tongue and mouth tissues; painful mouth and reduced appetite	Pupa in soil for 1–3 months; adult flies emerge in summer
Anoplocephela (tapeworm)	No migratory stage	Erosion of ileocaecal valve area; irritation to large intestine; loss of condition; occasional colic

through the body tissues and causing damage. Young horses are most vulnerable, because they have not been able to develop a natural tolerance to or immunity against the worms.

The extent of a worm infestation can be ascertained but it is not a simple exercise. A single faecal egg count simply reflects the presence of adult egg-laying worms. Regular faecal egg counts are more useful and these can be used to build up a picture of events occurring in each horse. More useful diagnoses are made using blood tests. These will confirm heavy worm burdens.

The most common worms affecting horses are shown in Table 13.3.

External parasites

Lice

There are two species of lice which affect horses, namely the sucking louse (*Haematopinus asini*) and the biting louse (*Damalina equi*) (Figure 13.6). The sucking louse feeds on the horse's blood, and the biting louse on scurf and debris on the skin surface.

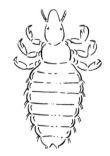

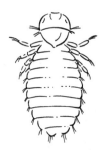

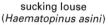

sucking louse
(*Haematopinus asini*)

biting louse
(*Damalina equi*)

Figure 13.6 The two species of lice that affect horses.

They are both small, grey, slow moving and easily overlooked. They are just visible to the naked eye (1.5–3 mm long). Their cream-coloured eggs, known as *nits*, are attached to the hair close to the root. They spend their entire life cycle, which is complete within three weeks, on the horse, which is their specific host. They do not live on humans. Lice cause severe itching, the coat becomes dull and scurfy and horses rapidly take on a moth-eaten appearance. Lice spread by direct contact and therefore all horses kept in the same field should be treated at the same time.

Flies

Flies are more of a nuisance than a true parasite even though some flies feed on horse's blood. They can be extremely irritating to horses, causing loss of condition, introduction of infections to wounds, eyes, etc., and also spread diseases from one horse to another. Sometimes flies can frighten horses, and this can lead to many problems and injuries, particularly in the summer months.

House flies (Musca domestica)

House flies are attracted to the moist parts of the body, such as the nose, eyes, vulva, prepuce and wounds. They may cause ulcerative dermatitis around the eyes. Although they do not bite, they can congregate in large numbers causing a high nuisance factor to the horse. Masks are available to prevent flies irritating the horse's eyes (Figure 13.7).

Stable flies (Stomoxys calcitrans)

Stable flies cause a considerable nuisance because, as well as sucking the horse's blood, their saliva may cause an allergic reaction. Unfortunately, they are widespread and abundant, breeding in bedding and

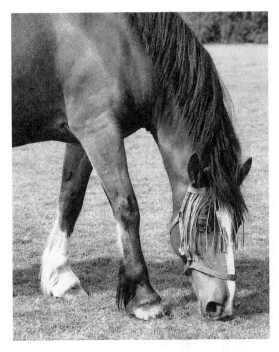

Figure 13.7

muck heaps. The bite is painful. The bite may leave raised swellings on the horse's skin and these flies will also bite humans.

Horse flies (Tabanus)

Horse flies have a particularly painful, deep bite. They have blade-like slashing mouth parts which create a pool of blood on which the fly feeds. They cause severe anxiety amongst horses, who will gallop around in order to escape from them. Horse flies also transmit the disease equine infectious anaemia.

Bot flies (Gasterophilus)

Bot flies lay their characteristic yellow eggs on the horse's front legs, chest and abdomen. Again, horses become very distressed when these flies are around. The larvae attach themselves to the stomach wall after having been swallowed by the horse.

Midges (Culicoides)

The biting midges are very small (0.5–3mm), hence their nickname 'no see-ums'. Many species bite and annoy horses, but only some species

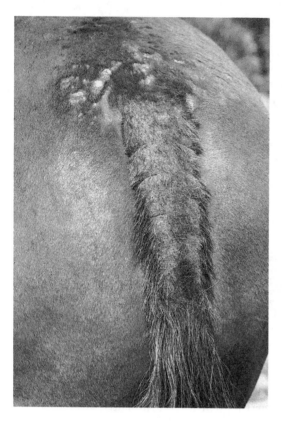

Figure 13.8 A horse severely affected by sweet itch.

cause the allergic reaction known as 'sweet itch' or *seasonal recurrent dermatitis*. Some horses have such severe reactions to the midges' saliva that they rub themselves raw on the mane and tail (Figure 13.8).

Summary points
• Bacteria are very small living cells • Viruses are not cells • Vaccination helps protect the horse from an infectious disease by exposing it to a mild or dead version of the micro-organism • Viruses replicate themselves by invading the nucleus of the horse's cells and using the horse's own DNA to make copies of itself • Bacteria damage the horse's cells and produce toxins • Some bacteria are necessary for the horse's health, e.g. hind-gut bacteria • Worms are internal parasites of the horse • Flies, ticks and lice are external parasites

Genetics and Heredity

14

The gene is the unit of heredity and is found in all organisms, plants and animals alike. Genes are passed from generation to generation, from parents to offspring, and are responsible for all aspects of an organism's make-up, from their cell and tissue structure and the processes within the body, to more visible traits such as the way they look and their size. For example, in horses, the presence of genes can be seen easily in characteristics such as breed, type, height, temperament and hair colour (Figure 14.1).

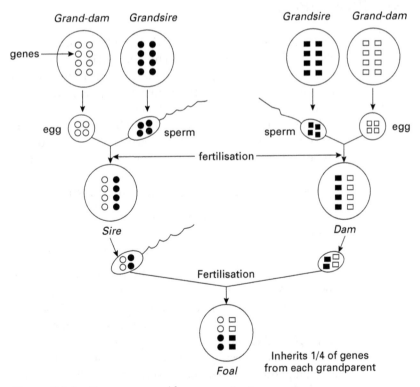

Figure 14.1 Genes are passed from generation to generation.

Table 14.1   Comparison of chromosome numbers in some organisms.

Organism	Diploid number of chromosomes
Horse	64
Human	46
Cat	38
Mouse	40
Pea	14
Barley	14
Maize	20
Fruit fly	8

Genes are located on chromosomes, which are found within the nucleus of cells. Each species has a specific number of chromosomes within the cell nucleus and this is known as the *diploid number*. Horses have 64 chromosomes whereas humans have 46 (Table 14.1). Chromosomes are arranged in pairs, known as *homologous chromosomes* or *homologous pairs*, so horses have 32 pairs and humans 23 pairs. One half of each pair is derived from each of the two parents.

THE STRUCTURE OF DNA

Genes consist of genetic material or DNA (deoxyribonucleic acid). DNA carries the genetic code. This code carries instructions for making proteins, which then go on to determine the function of an organism's cells and eventually the organism's final appearance.

Two scientists, Francis Crick and James Watson, unravelled the molecular structure of DNA in 1953. They were able to determine how the components of DNA fit together in a complex three-dimensional shape known as a double helix. This helix is composed of two strands, which are themselves made up of smaller units called nucleotides. Nucleotides have three parts making up their structure (Figure 14.2):

- A sugar known as a deoxyribose
- A phosphate group
- One of four bases: adenine, thymine, guanine and cytosine

The nucleotides are referred to by the initial letter of the base they carry, so A, T, G and C. The nucleotides are linked together in long strands known as polynucleotides. Each strand is made up of just these four nucleotides, repeated thousands of times. It is the sequence of A, T, G and C that makes up the genetic code.

Each DNA molecule consists of two of these polynucleotide strands joined together by weak bonds between each base, similar to the rungs of a ladder. These two strands are then twisted, giving the famous double helix structure of DNA. A DNA molecule is thought to carry

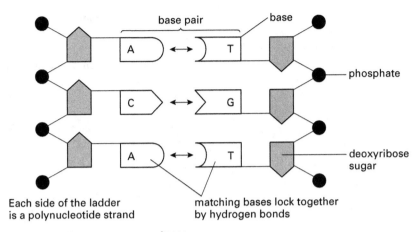

Each side of the ladder
is a polynucleotide strand

matching bases lock together
by hydrogen bonds

Figure 14.2 Basic structure of DNA.

approximately 1000 genes and each gene is a section of DNA of about 250 rungs of the ladder.

The bases have specific matches, so adenine can only bond with thymine and cytosine with guanine. Where an adenine occurs in one strand a thymine will be present opposite it on the other strand, and the same for cytosine and guanine. This pairing is important when DNA is copied, which happens when cells divide and multiply. An organism grows by cell division and each new cell receives a copy of the genetic code.

DNA REPLICATION

Before cell division, DNA must make a carbon copy of itself. To do this, the DNA helix structure unwinds under the influence of an enzyme. An enzyme splits the bonds connecting the bases. The two strands separate relatively easily and each one remains fully intact, rather like two halves of a zip. Another enzyme then attaches free nucleotides from within the cell to the now exposed bases on each of the two strands. This results in a carbon copy of the original DNA and the process is known as *replication*. Each new DNA molecule now contains one of the original polynucleotide strands and a new exact copy. The cell can now divide with this process ensuring that each new cell contains a complete copy of the original DNA.

Alleles

An allele is a form of a gene. Alleles are found at the same location or *locus* on homologous chromosomes and are separated during

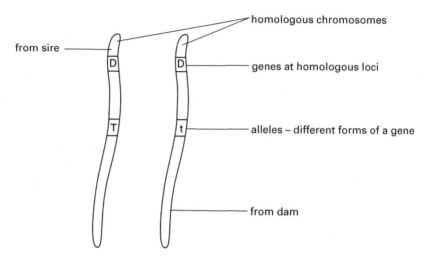

Figure 14.3 Alleles are found on homologous chromosomes at the same loci.

meiosis. Genes carried on pairs of homologous chromosomes are also paired and instruction sequences run down each homologous chromosome in the same order. Paired genes therefore control the same characteristic and may give identical instructions (Figure 14.3) or may also give slightly different instructions from each other. The different versions of the same gene (for a particular trait) are known as alleles.

Dominance

With a pair of alleles, one allele may be dominant to the other, in that it masks out the effect of the other allele in the pair. This is termed the dominant allele, and the other is termed the recessive allele. Sometimes one allele may not be completely dominant and this is known as *incomplete dominance* or *blending*. For example, a lack of dominance between a gene for red colour and one for white may result in a roan colour in horses. Codominance occurs when a pair of alleles controlling the same characteristic give different instructions but neither is dominant. The effects of both are represented in the result. An example of this is blood group in humans. The blood group AB results from codominance of the gene for the A group and the gene for the B group.

Gene regulation

All of the horse's cells contain the same genes within the chromosomes, but specific genes must be switched off or turned on. For example, genes to grow hooves are turned on in the coronary band, but are turned off everywhere else.

Cells therefore not only have a genetic programme for proteins but also a regulatory programme for expression of those genes.

Protein production

Part of the genetic information in DNA is devoted to the production of proteins which are essential to the horse's body and are used in a variety of ways. Proteins are made from templates of information in the DNA and are built up from long chains of amino acids in a set sequence. The sequence of the amino acids determines the structure and function of the protein. There are approximately 20 naturally-occurring amino acids. Genetic information required for protein synthesis is contained within the DNA in the nucleus of the cell, however protein manufacture takes place in the ribosomes and so information must be transferred from the nucleus to the ribosomes. This is done via messenger RNA (mRNA).

Sex cells

Sexual reproduction in all animals involves the fusion of one egg and one sperm, a process termed fertilisation. These sex cells are also known as gametes. Gametes are produced from cells that contain the full complement of chromosomes, called somatic cells. These divide to form two daughter cells but, unlike in normal cells, the DNA is not copied. Instead the paired chromosomes are divided equally, one of each pair going to each daughter cell. This process of division is called meiosis. These daughter cells (gametes) are termed haploid, which means they only contain half the number of chromosomes of the parent. This means that when the gametes fuse and fertilisation occurs, the offspring will receive half their DNA from the mother and half from the father.

The haploid number (the number of chromosomes in a gamete) is referred to as n, and the diploid number (the number of chromosomes in all cells other than gametes) is 2n. As we mentioned before, the diploid number for horses is 64, in humans it is 46.

HEREDITY

Horses vary even within the same breed. There may be differences in size, colour, bone, weight, condition, temperament, and even thickness of skin. These differences are known as variation. Variation may be:

Table 14.2   Examples of variation in horses.

Inherited	Environmental
Coat colour	Length of coat
Markings	Scars
Hoof colour	Length of hoof
Laryngeal paralysis (roaring/whistling)	COPD
Eye colour e.g. wall eye	

Height, Weight and Condition
(Genetic and environmental factors combine together)

- Genetic (inherited)
- Environmental, e.g. diet, surroundings, workload

Table 14.2 shows examples of variation in horses.

Genes will affect the range of heights and weights into which a horse or pony of a certain breed should fit, but environmental factors such as feeding will determine its position in the range.

During fertilisation, the gametes, containing half the genetic material of each parent, fuse and the resulting cell from which the offspring will develop now has a full set of chromosomes, the diploid number. This mixing of genes from two different individuals provides a completely new individual with their own unique genetic make-up, and it is this that provides genetic variation.

Sex determination

Horses have 32 pairs of chromosomes (a total of 64, as mentioned before). One pair is the sex chromosomes, and these carry the genes that determine the sex of the horse.

There are two sex chromosomes, X and Y. Females have two X chromosomes denoted XX, males have an X and a Y, denoted XY. Therefore eggs from the mother will only carry an X chromosome but the sperm from the father may carry either an X or a Y chromosome because the father has both chromosomes in his genetic make-up and when his somatic cells divide to form gametes, half will receive an X and half will receive a Y. Therefore, a foal's sex is determined by the genetic information it receives from the sire at fertilisation. At fertilisation, the sperm may be an X or a Y. If the egg is fertilised by a sperm containing a Y, the offspring will be a colt whereas if it is fertilised by a sperm containing an X, the foal will be a filly.

Table 14.3 Sex determination

SIRE = XY
DAM = XX

	SIRE X chromosome	SIRE Y chromosome
DAM X chromosome	XX filly	XY colt
DAM X chromosome	XX filly	XY colt

To summarise:

- Colts inherit an X from the dam and a Y from the sire
- Fillies inherit an X from the dam and an X from the sire

Figure 14.3 shows how sex determination works. The diagram is known as a punnet square. This is used to work out the predicted genetic result of the random crossing of the gametes. The sire's characteristics are listed on the top and the dam's on the side of the punnet square.

Genotype and phenotype

Genotype refers to the genetic makeup of the animal, whereas phenotype refers to the animal's appearance. Phenotype is a result of both genotype and environment.

Monohybrid inheritance

Gregor Johann Mendel (1822–1884) was an Augustinian monk who carried out numerous experiments on pea plants. He noticed that these plants showed two basic colours, white and red. When white pea plants were pollinated with red pea plants the resultant plants of this first generation, known as F1, had only red flowers. When he crossed these red-flowered plants with each other to produce a second generation (F2), a few of the resulting plants had white flowers. So two red-flowered plants had produced white-flowered offspring. He realised that the code for white was recessive to red, so the first generation only showed red flowers, but they must still contain the instructions for white flowers. Although at that time DNA, genes and alleles had not been discovered, Mendel had worked out that some of the gametes from the F1 generation must carry the recessive allele for white flowers, and if they fertilise a gamete which also contains a recessive allele then the F2 generation would have some white-flowered individuals, despite red being the dominant colour.

From his experiments he formulated two basic laws of inheritance, these are known as Mendel's Laws or Mendelian Inheritance:

- Law of segregation – the alleles of a gene separate into different gametes
- Law of independent assortment – the female gamete may be fertilised by any male gamete

This is simple inheritance, each parent contributing one allele to the offspring. Alleles as discussed previously, are found at the same loci and affect the same trait. Simple dominance refers to two alleles at one locus where one masks the effects of the other. The effects of the recessive allele are 'masked' by those of the dominant one.

Another example of simple dominance is the black coat colour in horses. As discussed in Chapter 8, horses may manufacture two basic pigments within the hair. These are:

- Eumelanin (black pigment)
- Phaeomelanin (red pigment)

Black coat colour in horses is dominant to red. Red is therefore said to be recessive to black. The dominant black allele allows the horse to produce eumelanin in addition to phaeomelanin. The recessive allele allows the horse to produce only phaeomelanin, in this case resulting in a red coat colour, which is only shown in the absence of the dominant black allele.

When two recessive traits such as red and red are crossed with each other, the resultant offspring will always be red and this is known as 'breeding true'. The two primary alleles at the E or extension locus are E and e. The dominant gene for black is referred to as E for eumelanin and phaeomelanin. The recessive allele is referred to as e for phaeomelanin.

For these alleles for black, the following gentoypes and phenotypes result.

Genotype EE – Phenotype black hair
Genotype Ee – Phenotype black hair
Genotype ee – Phenotype red hair

Where both alleles are the same e.g. EE or ee, the horse is said to be *homozygous* for that trait. Where they are different such as Ee, the horse is said to be *heterozygous* for the trait.

A punnet square can be used to predict what may happen when a heterozygous black sire is crossed with a heterozygous black mare.

		From sire	
		E	e
From dam	E	EE black	Ee black
	e	Ee black	ee red

The result is one homozygous dominant black EE, two heterozygous black Ee and one red ee.

There will be three black foals to one red foal i.e. the phenotype ratio will be 3:1.

Test cross or back cross

To find out whether a dominant phenotype is from the homozygous EE or the heterozygous Ee, then a test cross can be carried out with a homozygous ee or red phenotype.

The following results are expected.

		From sire	
		E	e
From dam	e	Ee black	ee red
	e	Ee black	ee red

The resultant ratio is 1:1, one black to one red.

A review of the family history of a group of horses can help to determine probable genotypes from their phenotypes. For example a black horse that produces a chestnut foal must be heterozygous Ee and a black foal from a chestnut parent will also be Ee.

Dihybrid inheritance

This refers to inheritance of two pairs of characteristics. In this example, black coat colour and height are used.

T is tall and dominant and t is short and recessive
E is black and dominant and e is red and recessive

This cross refers to a tall black mare TTEE and a short red sire ttee.
Meiosis results in the following gametes:

TE   TE   te   te

		From sire	
		te	te
From dam	TE	TtEe tall black	TtEe tall black
	TE	TtEe tall black	TtEe Tall black

The F1 offspring are all tall black foals!

If two of the F1 offspring are crossed the following results.
Meiosis results in the following gametes:

TE   Te   te   te

		From sire			
		TE	Te	tE	te
From dam	TE	TTEE tall black	TTEe tall black	TtEE tall black	TtEe tall black
	Te	TTEe tall black	TTee tall red	TtEe tall black	Ttee tall red
	tE	TtEE tall black	TtEe tall black	ttEE short black	ttEe short black
	te	TtEe tall black	Ttee tall red	ttEe short black	ttee short red

The F2 offspring foals are:

9 tall black foals
3 tall red foals
3 short black foals
1 short red foal

It was from this type of dihybrid cross that Mendel formulated the law
of independent assortment.

Epistasis and hypostasis

Sometimes the presence of a certain allele at a locus may affect the expression of a gene at a completely different locus. This is not to be confused with dominance, which refers to the effects of alleles of a single gene. When there is a certain combination of alleles at a locus (the epistatic locus), the expression of the genotype at another locus (the hypostatic locus) will be masked.

A good example of epistasis may be seen with black, chestnut and bay colours. All horses have a basic colour of black, chestnut or bay before the modification of colour and patterning occurs from other genes.

Polygenic or multiple gene traits

Most traits are the result of more than one gene working together. An example of a polygenic trait is blue eye colour and white markings in horses, and also conformation traits. The exact genetic mechanism of this polygenic inheritance is unknown.

Sex linkage

Some traits are sex linked if the sex chromosome pair is involved. If a female has a defective gene on one of her two X chromosomes, she will be protected from its effects by the normal gene on her second X chromosome. If a male has a mutant X and a normal Y chromosome, he will be affected by a X-linked disease. The X and Y chromosomes are so-called because of their shapes and the Y chromosome is much smaller than the X chromosome, containing much less genetic information. This can result in the X chromosome having no pair on the Y chromosome. If there is no pair on the Y chromosome then the allele on the X chromosome will express itself in the male because there is no 'partner' conferring an effect from the Y chromosome. Alleles found on only the X chromosome are known as sex-linked alleles.

An example of sex linkage is found in the condition haemophilia, where the blood fails to clot properly during bleeding. The alleles are as follows:

X_H – normal allele
X_h – allele for haemophilia

Females can be haemophiliac (X_hX_h) but this is very rare. Females can carry the haemophilia allele on one of their X chromosomes (X_HX_h) but they will not fully develop the condition because they have two X chromosomes and so have another normally functioning allele.

		From sire	
		X$_H$	Y
From dam	X$_H$	X$_H$X$_H$ normal female	X$_H$Y normal male
	Xh	X$_H$Xh carrier female	XhY haemophiliac male

Lethal genes

Genes may cause a lethal condition and these are therefore known as lethal genes. There are several lethal genes in horses. Most lethal genes only have the lethal effect when the horse is homozygous for the mutant allele. The heterozygotes are therefore known as carriers for the lethal condition.

An example of a lethal gene in horses is the Lethal White. The affected foals are born white or mostly white with a condition termed atresia coli. This is an incomplete development of the large colon and the foal cannot defecate.

Genetic variation

There are two types of genetic variation:

- Continuous variation
- Discontinuous variation

Continuous variation

Genes that code for characteristics such as body weight and height display continuous variation, in that within a group an animal can have any weight or height. Horses can be any weight or height within a large range, for example Shetlands are very small (Figure 14.4), other breeds e.g. the shire are much larger. The characteristics are controlled by many genes and are therefore known as polygenic.

Discontinuous variation

This refers to distinct forms of a characteristic, such as eye colour or blood group.

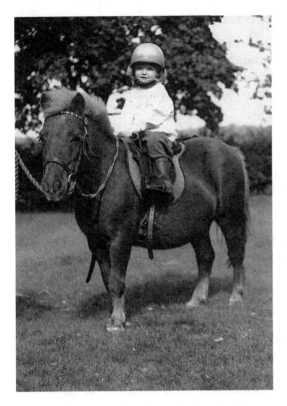

Figure 14.4   Shetland pony.

Causes of variation

There are several influences causing variation. These include:

- Environmental influences
- Genetic influences

Environmental influences

The environmental conditions to which an animal is exposed may produce differences in appearance. This can be seen in identical twins where environmental effects such as diet, or ill health may result in appearance differences.

Genetic influences

- Gene recombination
- Mutation

The process of sexual reproduction produces variation by:

- Cross-fertilisation, the genes of the two parents are mixed
- During meiosis, the random distribution of chromosomes on the spindle, followed by separation leads to further mixing of genes
- Crossing over between homologous chromosomes during meiosis recombines linked genes

Mutation

Mutation is a change to the DNA or chromosomes, and can affect the structure or information contained in the genetic material. Only mutations which arise in the formation of the sex cells or gametes are inherited. The rate of mutation is slow, but external factors such as radiation or chemicals may increase the rate of mutation. These are known as mutagenic factors.

Mutations tend to be random. Some may be beneficial, giving an advantage to an organism. Darwin proposed that this is the mechanism for evolution. A mutation that gives an organism an advantage over others means that it will be more likely to survive and pass on its genes, so the mutation is passed on and becomes more common within the group. Eventually, over many millions of years, groups diverge and form new species.

Other mutations may be lethal and will therefore not be passed on to future generations. Some mutations may not be lethal but put an animal at a disadvantage and so organisms that have that trait are less likely to pass on their genetic material.

Gene mutation

These occur due to a change in the DNA at a single locus on the chromosome, for example a nucleotide may be mis-copied so instead of an A there is now a T or one nucleotide might be missed out when the DNA is copied. Such mutations may or may not have an effect on the organism.

Chromosome mutation

Sometimes chromosomes fail to separate properly during meiosis and this results in the gamete having the diploid number (2n) of chromosomes instead of the necessary haploid number (n). If this gamete fuses with another normal haploid sex cell, then the resultant embryo will be triploid in number, i.e. 3n. This is known as polyploidy.

During meiosis other errors can occur, such as chromosomes being lost from a gamete, being damaged or their structure altered.

Selective breeding

For many years, breeders have tried to breed horses with special characteristics such as speed or conformation. This is known as artifical selection. Artificial selection is carried out as follows:

- Select the best sire and dam
- Breed them
- Take the best offspring
- Breed from them

All thoroughbred racehorses can be traced back to three Arab horses. This has reduced the number of different alleles and thus the potential variation available for breeding in the future.

Cloning

A clone is an organism that is genetically identical to another organism. The first mammal to be cloned was a sheep known as 'Dolly' in 1995. Recently, claims have been made that the first horse has been cloned. Dolly was cloned when a cell was taken from an adult sheep (in this case from the udder but any cell would do). At the same time an egg was taken from the ovary of another sheep and its nucleus removed. The egg was then fused with the adult cell from the udder and placed in the uterus of another ewe which served as the surrogate mother. From this process Dolly was born.

Animals may also be cloned by the splitting of an embryo. The early embryo contains a ball of identical stem cells, each of which is capable of developing into a new individual. Splitting an early embryo therefore results in two identical individuals (identical twins).

Genetic engineering

Genes control the production of all proteins. Genetic engineering involves taking a specific gene from one organism and placing it in another. This enables the new organism to make protein it was not able to make before. The organism which receives the new genetic material as known as a genetically-modified organism (GMO).

Genetic engineering has several advantages:

- It is much faster than conventional plant and animal breeding programmes that seek to change particular traits over several generations
- Genes may be transferred between any types of organism
- Cheaper manufacture of some important drugs or hormones such as insulin

GM crops are already produced that are resistant to some pests, herbicides and disease. Genetic engineering has helped scientists produce useful chemicals in a fast and efficient way. One example is the hormone insulin. This hormone is important for lowering blood glucose levels and is normally produced in the pancreas. Some humans, due to a condition known as diabetes, are not able to make enough insulin and therefore it must be given by injection. Historically, human insulin has been made for diabetic patients by extraction from the pancreas of pigs and cows following slaughter. This is an expensive and long-winded process which results in animal insulin and not human. This also has ethical implications for diabetics who do not wish to use animal insulin.

Now, the gene which makes human insulin, has been identified. This gene has been removed from human cells, copied and then placed within bacterial cells. The bacteria multiply rapidly and start producing insulin. Genetically-engineered insulin has been made this way for over twenty years.

GM FOODS

GM or genetically-modified foods are now available. Plants are genetically engineered or modified to help make them more resistant to pests or herbicides. The genetic moderations are minor and as such pose little risk to the health of the animal eating the food. Genetically-modified soya oil is indistinguishable from conventional soya oil. However, there has been much controversy regarding the use of GM foods and many horse-feed companies now pronounce their ranges of feeds as GM-free. Producers of GM foods fully research and analyse the products, checking for any problems. It is the responsibility of the manufacturer to make sure that GM foods are safe.

Concerns regarding the safety of GM crops include:

- Transfer of genes through GM foods to other animals including humans
- Cross-pollination with other crops or weeds
- Toxicity for pests also affecting other useful animals

Firstly, one of a few genes from a GM crop may be attached to the transferred gene that once within the body may create problems of its own.

All cells within new genetically-modified organisms will contain the new gene. For plants, this will include pollen. So GM plants, once flowered, may spread to other fields and pollinate non-GM plants growing there. Pollen may be dispersed over wide areas, for example by wind and insects. This is a particular concern for organic farmers who pride themselves on the natural quality of their crops.

GM plants that are resistant to specific herbicides may cross-pollinate wild plants, resulting in weeds that are now modified to be resistant to herbicides. GM crops that have been made to be toxic to certain pests may also be toxic to useful insects or other animals and this may affect the ecology of the field. Also, animals such as insects that have eaten the GM crop may not be affected but may now be carrying the gene. Another animal higher in the food chain that perhaps eats one of these insects will take in this gene and this could cause problems.

This has implications for the horse industry for both grazing animals and feeding GM crops.

Summary points

- A gene is the unit of heredity and is made of DNA.
- Alleles or variations of genes exist, which may have slightly different effects in the organism. One allele may have an effect that masks the effect of its paired allele. This masking is termed dominance, so the allele is the dominant allele. The masked allele is termed recessive.
- DNA codes for all the proteins in a horse's body.
- The parent has the full complement of chromosomes, the diploid number. In horses this is 64. The parent's gametes, formed by meiosis, contain only half that amount, the haploid number. In horses this is 32. This means that when two gametes, one from each parent, fuse, the offspring then has the full complement of chromosomes.
- Males have XY and the female XX chromosomes.
- Some traits are sex linked.
- Mutation is a change in the DNA structure. This may not have an effect, it may be advantageous or disadvantageous and is a way in which variety can occur in a species.

Teeth and Estimating Age

Horses have evolved to graze little and often and their teeth have evolved along with them. Each tooth has a crown that is high in relation to the length of the root, a condition known as *hypsodont*, whereas humans have low-crowned, or *brachydont*, teeth (Figure 15.1). In horses, most of the crown protrudes below the gum line (the root is deep), but the tooth grows continuously so that tooth wear is compensated for by tooth growth. They continue to grow and wear down until the horse is 20–30 years of age. During this time, changes occur in the shape and patterns of the teeth that allow knowledgeable people to gauge a horse's age.

The modern horse has fewer teeth than its ancestors, and has lost the first pair of premolar teeth. These sometimes reappear as *vestigial* (functionless), or 'wolf' teeth, in young male horses.

Like humans, horses have two sets of teeth during their lifetime: the temporary (*deciduous*) 'milk' teeth and the permanent adult teeth.

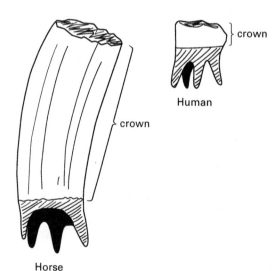

crown

Human

crown

Horse

Figure 15.1 Comparison of the human and equine tooth.

The temporary teeth are smaller and whiter then the adult teeth, but there are no temporary or baby molars. From the age of about two and half years, the temporary teeth are gradually replaced by the adult permanent teeth, until there is a full set of these at about five years of age.

Types of teeth

Horses have three types of teeth (Figure 15.2):

- *Incisors* – front biting teeth
- *Molars* and *premolars* – cheek teeth used for grinding (Figure 15.3); unlike those of humans, in horses the molars and premolars are very similar in shape
- *Canines* – tushes (in males and 25% of mares)

Incisors are used for tearing and cutting grass. The horse's incisors may be seen in Figure 15.4.

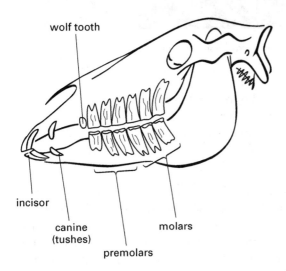

Figure 15.2 Tooth position in horses.

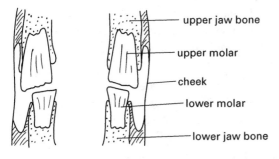

Figure 15.3 Cross-section of the molar teeth, front view.

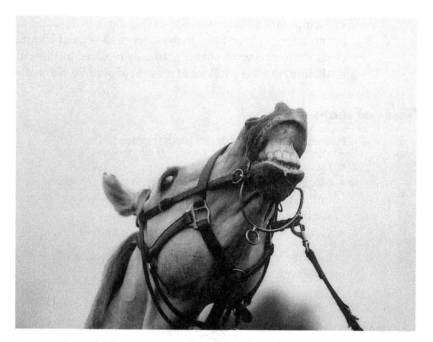

Figure 15.4   This horse's incisors may be seen clearly.

The incisors are further divided into:

- *Centrals* – the pair top and bottom in the centre
- *Laterals* – the teeth next to the centrals
- *Corners* – teeth next to the laterals

Dental formulae

Young horses have a total number of 24 temporary teeth – 12 incisors and 12 premolars or grinding teeth. Mature male horses have 40–42 permanent teeth while mares have 36–40 depending upon the presence or absence of canine teeth. Mares have canine teeth 20–25% of the time and these are usually smaller than those found in males. The first premolar or wolf tooth may be rudimentary or absent altogether. In most horses it is seen only in the upper jaw. Canine teeth tend to erupt in the interdental space at 4–5 years of age in male horses.

The dental formulae for mature males and mares are shown in the diagrams below (for simplicity, only one side of the mouth is shown, but the left and right sides are the same).

Male	Female
(2) × 3.1.3 or 4.3 = 40–42	(2) × 3.0.3 or 4.3 = 36–40
3.1.3.3	3.0.3.3
I.C.P.M.	I.C.P.M.

I – Incisors, C – Canine, P – Premolars, M – Molars

Table 15.1 Age of appearance of temporary and permanent teeth.

Tooth	Temporary ('milk') teeth	Permanent (adult) teeth
Incisors		
First	Birth–1 week of age	2.5 years
Second	4–6 weeks	3.5 years
Third	6–9 months	4.5 years
Canines (tushes)	n/a	from 4–5 years
Premolars		
First	Birth–2 weeks	5–6 months
Second	same	2.5 years
Third	same	3 years
Fourth	same	3.5 years
Molars		
First	n/a	9–12 months
Second	n/a	2 years
Third	n/a	from 3.5–4 years

Table 15.1 shows the appearance times of temporary and permanent teeth.

Tooth structure

Each tooth consists of three layers (Figure 15.5):

- *Dentine* – hard substance similar to bone; contains calcium; found in the centre of the tooth
- *Enamel* – porcelain-like covering of the tooth; one of the hardest substances in the horse's body
- *Cement* – covers the crown of the tooth; bone-like; cushions the root, preventing it from becoming brittle

Wear of the tooth

Grass contains one of the hardest known substances, namely silica. (Silica is used to make glass!) Repeated chewing, in a side to side and a circular motion, works the ingested grass material into a wad. This wad is passed further back down, to the premolars and molars, which continue to grind it down, before swallowing it. This continuous chewing of forage causes excessive wear of the teeth.

New permanent teeth have a large crown, much of which is situated below the gum line. In the five-year-old horse, the last three or four molars in the upper jaw fill as far back as the maxillary sinus, reaching above the facial crest level. As the tooth wears down from grazing, the root pushes the crown up to compensate. By the time the horse is

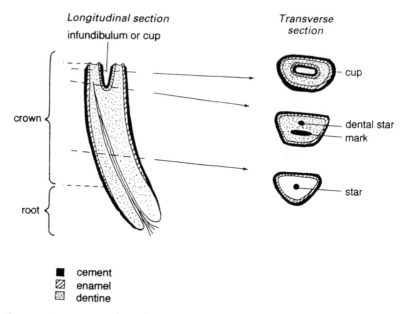

Longitudinal section

infundibulum or cup

*Transverse
section*

cup

dental star
mark

crown

star

root

■ cement
▨ enamel
▩ dentine

Figure 15.5 Section through an incisor tooth, showing its structure.

twelve years of age, the roots are no longer distinct, are closed up and the teeth occupy less space within the jaw. As horses continue to age, there is less and less crown embedded in the jaw until it has all been pushed up and the tooth is eventually lost.

As the biting surface of the tooth is worn away, the pattern on the tooth table changes. The cement is worn away first, exposing the enamel, which is then worn away to expose the dentine. Soon after the tooth has come into wear, five rings of cement, enamel and dentine surround the cup or *infundibulum*.

The cement and dentine wear away first, leaving the enamel standing proud in ridges. These ridges provide a table that is highly effective for grinding down forage material. As the tooth table wears further, the cup becomes shallower until all that remains is a mark or enamel surrounding cement. This mark is a long oval shape, which gradually becomes a smaller rounded spot as further wear takes place.

When eventually the pulp cavity is reached, it appears on the tooth as a *dental star*. (As the tooth wears down, the sensitive tissues, such as nerves, are protected by a secondary layer of dentine seen on the tooth table as the dental star.) For a short time both the spot and the dental star are visible, the spot or mark lying behind the dental star. As the horse ages, the dental star becomes more central and rounded.

The horse's teeth also change with age in shape, becoming more triangular, and in angulation, becoming less upright.

DETERMINING AGE BY DENTITION (AGEING)

The changes in appearance of the teeth are used to 'age' horses. Generally the lower incisor teeth are used, with the patterns on the teeth, their angulation and shape all being taken into account.

Horses fall into three distinct age groups for ageing:

- Birth to five years of age – use eruption and wear of adult teeth
- 5–12 years of age – use the pattern on the tooth table
- 12 years and older (aged horses) – dentition less reliable for ageing

Figure 15.6 shows how a horse's age may be assessed from its tooth pattern. It is important to note that this is not an exact science – Galvayne's groove, for example, may not always be present.

Ageing the young horse

Ageing the young horse will depend upon the eruption of both temporary and permanent teeth. By the time the foal is one year old it will have a full mouth of temporary incisor teeth. It takes six months from the time of eruption for an incisor tooth to grow to meet its partner tooth on the opposing jaw and come into wear. At 12 months of age, the centrals and laterals are in wear, but not the corners.

Two year olds have a full set of temporary incisor teeth that are all in wear. At about two and a half years of age, the central incisor teeth are replaced by permanent teeth, so that at three years of age the adult centrals are erupted and in wear. These teeth will look more yellow, because of their cement covering, and larger than the temporary teeth.

At about three and a half years, the adult teeth replace the lateral incisors, so that by age four the permanent centrals and laterals are in wear. At about four and a half years, the adult corner incisors erupt so that the five year old has a full set of permanent teeth. Also during this time, the molars and premolars have been developing, although these are not used for ageing horses. It should be remembered that the centrals are a year older than the laterals, which are a year older than the corners.

The young horse does not have any temporary molar teeth, because the foal's jaws are not big enough to house them. By the time the foal is three months of age, it will have three pairs of temporary premolars on each side of the jaw. The first permanent molar appears behind these premolars at about 9–12 months of age. At two and a half the first permanent premolars appear and the other two are replaced at three and a half. The final molar tooth erupts at four and half years of age. These changes can result in a lumpy appearance to the young horse's lower jaw. Once the horse has a 'full mouth', the age is then estimated by the changing patterns on the tooth table.

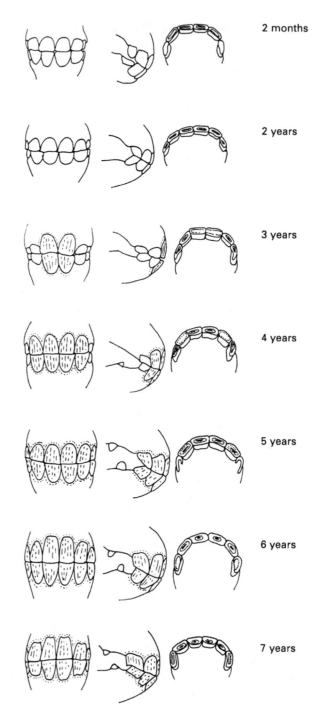

Figure 15.6   Ageing horses from their teeth.

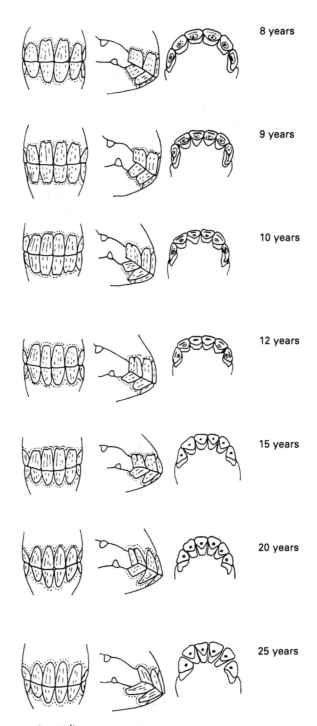

8 years

9 years

10 years

12 years

15 years

20 years

25 years

Figure 15.6   (cont'd)

Ageing the 6–12 year old

The six year old will have all the incisors in wear, with level tables showing a dark cup. In the seven year old, the cup in the central incisors will have worn out leaving the 'mark', which is not as dark as the cup. The mark consists of an outline of enamel surrounding cement.

By eight years of age, the cup will have worn out of the laterals, leaving a mark, and the centrals will now have a dental star near the front of the tooth.

By nine years of age, the cup will have worn out of the corners, leaving a mark and the dental star will be apparent on the laterals. Galvayne's groove appears as a dark groove on the upper corner teeth at 9–10 years of age (Figure 15.7).

The ten year old will have stars and marks in all incisor teeth, and the stars will be clearer. The laterals will have rounded off to become more triangular in shape. Galvayne's groove then gradually grows down the tooth.

The twelve year old will have only dental stars in the centrals and the teeth are more triangular.

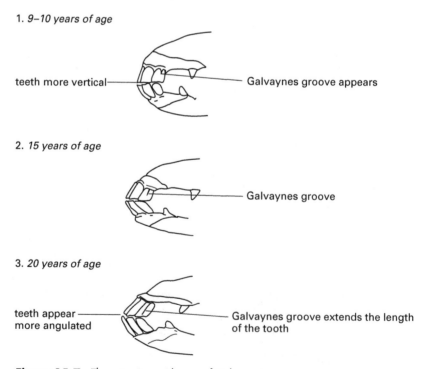

1. *9–10 years of age*

teeth more vertical —————— Galvaynes groove appears

2. *15 years of age*

Galvaynes groove

3. *20 years of age*

teeth appear more angulated —————— Galvaynes groove extends the length of the tooth

Figure 15.7 The extension, with age, of Galvayne's groove.

Ageing the older horse

The fifteen year old will only have dental stars on the tooth tables, and the teeth will have increased in slope i.e. they will be less vertical. Galvayne's groove now extends about halfway down the corner incisor.

By the time the horse is twenty years of age, Galvayne's groove will extend down the whole tooth.

Summary points

- Horses have high-crowned (hypsodont) teeth
- Modern horses have fewer teeth than their ancestors
- Young horses have a total of 24 temporary teeth
- Each tooth consists of three layers, dentine, enamel and cement
- Tooth wear enables the age of a horse to be estimated

Appendix 1 Useful Terms

Anatomy – study of the structure of the body
Physiology – study of how the parts of the body work
Pathology – study of abnormalities and how they cause ill health
Histology – study of cells and tissues
Microbiology – study of micro-organisms
Genetics – study of genes and heredity

ANATOMICAL TERMS

Anterior – in front of
Posterior – behind

Superficial – near the surface of the body
Deep – deeper within the body

Sagittal – in the dorsoventral plane

Caudal – towards the tail
Cranial – towards the head, surrounding the brain or between the ears

Dorsal – towards the horse's back
Ventral – towards the horse's belly

Plantar – part of lower limb facing forward
Palmar – part of lower limb facing backward

Distal – further away from the body
Proximal – closer to the body

Lateral – towards the side of the body
Medial – towards the midline of the body

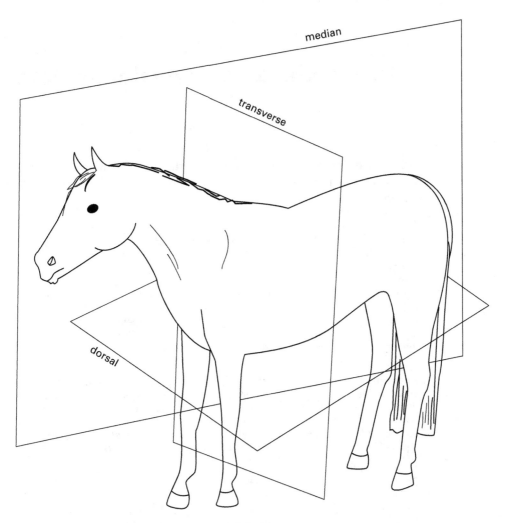

Median – in the middle – divides body into left & right
Dorsal – (frontal) – parallel to dorsal surface
Transverse – perpendicular to the body's long axis

Appendix 2   Conversion Factors

Below are some useful conversion factors. To change *to* metric, *multiply* by the figure shown. To change *from* metric, *divide* by the figure shown.

Imperial	Symbol	Conversion Factor	Metric	Symbol
Length				
miles	mi	1.6093	kilometres	km
yards	yd	0.9144	metres	m
feet	ft	0.3048	metres	m
inches	in	2.54	centimetres	cm
inches	in	25.4	millimetres	mm
furlong	fu	200	metres	m
Area				
square miles	mi^2	2.59	square kilometres	km^2
square miles	mi^2	258.999	hectares	ha
acres	acre	4046.86	square metres	m^2
acres	acre	0.4047	hectares	ha
square yards	yd^2	0.8361	square metres	m^2
square feet	ft^2	0.0929	square metres	m^2
Volume (liquid)				
gallons	gal	4.546	litres	l
pints	pint	0.568	litres	l
ounces	oz	28.41	millilitres	ml
teaspoon	tsp	5	millilitres	ml
Velocity				
miles per hour	mph	1.6093	kilometres per hour	kph
feet per second	fps	0.3048	metres per second	mps
Mass (weight)				
tons	ton	1.016	tonne	tonne
tons	ton	1016.05	kilograms	kg
pounds	lb	0.4536	kilograms	kg
ounces	oz	28.3495	grams	g

Some other useful equivalents

Multiply to change to the units on the *right*. *Divide* to change to the units on the *left*.

Change value from/to	Symbol	Conversion factor	Change value from/to	Symbol
ppm	mg/kg	0.001	ppm	mg/g
kilocalories	Kcal	4.1855	kilojoules	kJ
megacalories	Mcal	1000	kilocalories	Kcal
total digestible nutrients (TDN)	TDN/kg	4409	kilocalories	Kcal/kg
total digestible nutrients (TDN)	TDN/lb	2000	kilocalories	Kcal/lb
starch equivalent (SE)	SE/lb	2305	kilocalories	Kcal/lb
starch equivalent (SE)	SE/kg	5082	kilocalories	Kcal/kg
grams per kilogram	g/kg	0.1	percent	%
milligrams per kilogram	mg/kg	0.0001	percent	%
centigrade (Celsius)	°C	5/9 (°F–32)	Fahrenheit	°F
Fahrenheit	°F	9/5 (°C+32)	centigrade	°C
miles per hour	mph	88	feet per minute	fpm

Additional useful values

1 litre (l) = 1.7597 Imperial pints (pt)
1 mile (mi) = 8 furlongs (fu)
1 furlong (fu) = 200 metres (m)
1 hand = 4 inches (in)
1 mile (mi) = 5280 feet (ft)
1 kilogram (kg) = 2.2046 pounds (lb)
1 tonne = 1000 kg or 2200 pounds (lb)
1 Imperial ton = 907.18 kg or 2000 pounds (lb)

US and Imperial liquid measures

1 Imperial pint (pt) = 20 ounces (oz) = 568.26 millilitres (ml)
1 Imperial ounce = 28.4130 millilitres
1 US pint = 16 ounces = 473.176 millilitres
1 US ounce = 29.5735 millilitres

SI metric units and their symbols

Measurement of	SI unit	Symbol
Length	metre	m
Mass	kilogram	kg
Energy	joule	J

Metric unit prefixes

Prefix	Symbol	Multiple
mega-	M	10^6
kilo-	k	10^3
hecto-	h	10^2
deca-	da	10^1
deci-	d	10^{-1}
centi-	c	10^{-2}
milli-	m	10^{-3}
micro-	μ	10^{-6}
nano-	n	10^{-9}
pico-	p	10^{-12}

Therefore:

1 milligram (mg) is one thousandth of a gram (g) and 1 g = 1000 mg
1 microgram (μg) is one millionth of a gram (g) and 1 mg = 1000 μg

Units of vitamins

Vitamin	Metric	International Units (IU)
vitamin A	800 mcg	2400
vitamin D	5 mcg	200
vitamin E	10 mg	15

Appendix 3   Normal Diagnostic Values

Heart rate (pulse rate)
30–40 beats per minute
Respiration rate
8–12 breaths per minute
Temperature
38 °C (100.5 °F)
Blood pH
7.35–7.45

Blood tests – reference values

Haematology	Normal values
Red blood cells	$6.5–12.3 \times 10^{12}$/l
Haemoglobin	11.2–16.2 g/100ml
Packed cell volume (PCV)	34–44%
Total white blood cells	6000–12,000/mm^3
Total platelets	$200–400 \times 10^9$/l
Lymphocytes	$1.6–5.4 \times 10^9$/l
Neutrophils	$2.5–7.0 \times 10^9$/l
Monocytes	$0.6–0.7 \times 10^9$/l
Eosinophils	$0.0–0.3 \times 10^9$/l
Biochemistry	
Total albumin	25–41 g/l
Total globulin	25–41 g/l
Urea	3.5–7.3 mmol/l
Aspartate aminotransferase (AST/SGOT)	<250 U/l
Creatine kinase (CK/CPK)	<150 U/l
Gammaglutamyl transferase (GGT)	<40 U/l

Appendix 4   The Nitrogen Cycle

Scientists are able to assess the way in which many elements pass through living animals during their lifetime before becoming available again for use. This information is illustrated as *nutrient cycles*, perhaps the most important of which is the nitrogen cycle, which is shown below:

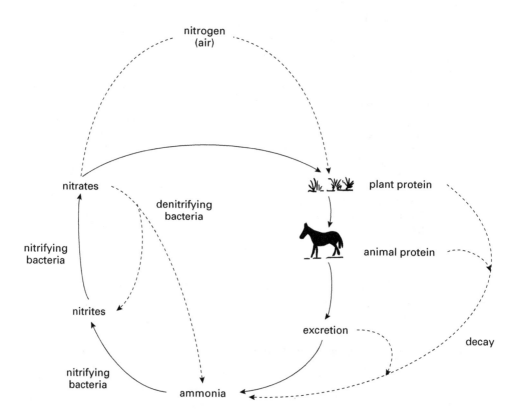

Appendix 5   Points of the Horse

The diagram below illustrates the points of the horse.

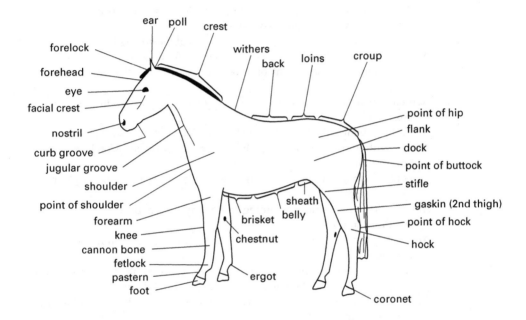

Glossary

ADP (Adenosine diphosphate) – substance found in all cells; converted to ATP during respiration

ATP (Adenosine triphosphate) – a high-energy compound used by all cells to store energy made from respiration

Absorption – uptake of substances into the cells of the horse's body

Acidosis – abnormally low blood pH caused by an excess of hydrogen ions

Active transport – movement of substances across a cell membrane using energy

Aerobic respiration – the release of energy from respiration in the presence of oxygen

Alkalosis – abnormally high blood pH caused by a lack of hydrogen ions

Alleles – different forms of a gene that occupy the same locus on homologous chromosomes

Alveolus – small air sac in the lung where gaseous exchange takes place (plural: alveoli)

Amino acids – molecules containing carbon, hydrogen, oxygen, nitrogen and sometimes sulphur

Anaerobic respiration – the release of energy from respiration in the absence of oxygen

Antibodies – proteins made by white blood cells that attach themselves to foreign cells or bodies (antigens) and help to destroy them

Aorta – the main artery of the body; carries oxygenated blood from the heart to the rest of the body

Articulation – the movement of two bones at a joint

Assimilation – the incorporation of absorbed food into various parts of the horse's body

Atrium – one of the two upper chambers of the heart (plural: atria)

Axon – a long process emerging from a nerve cell body that carries nervous impulses away from it

Base – a substance that reacts with an acid, neutralising it

Bile – An alkaline fluid made in the liver that passes into the duodenum aiding the digestion of fats

Bile salts – substances found in bile that help to emulsify fats

Bolus – a ball of food formed after chewing, which is then swallowed

Bronchiole – narrow air tube within the lungs, which is a subdivision of a bronchus

Bronchus – one of two wide tubes carrying air into the lung, a subdivision of the trachea (plural: bronchi)

Buffer – a chemical system that helps to maintain a constant pH

Caecum – a highly-developed part of the horse's digestive tract; used for cellulose digestion

Capillary – a tiny blood vessel, with walls that are one cell thick, enabling exchange of substances within the tissues

Carbohydrate – a substance made of carbon, hydrogen and oxygen, where the ratio of hydrogen to oxygen atoms is 2:1, e.g. sugars and starches

Carpus – 'knee' joint of the forelimb

Carpal bone – one of the bones in the horse's knee

Cartilage – a firm and flexible tissue used in movement and support

Catalyst – a substance that increases the rate of a chemical reaction but remains itself unchanged at the end of the reaction

Cell membrane – a very thin layer of protein and fat, which surrounds the protoplasm of all cells; membranes also line some organelles within the cell

Cellulose – a carbohydrate that is a major component of all plant cell walls; a polysaccharide formed from β-glucose

Centromere – the point at which two chromatids are joined during the early stages of cell division; where the spindle attaches

Cerebellum – the area of the brain that controls muscular co-ordination

Cerebrum – the part of the brain that controls conscious thought

Chromatid – one of two chromosome strands visible during prophase of mitosis

Chromosome – a coiled thread of DNA and protein found within the cell's nucleus

Cilia – small hair-like structures projecting from some cells

Cochlea – a coiled tube within the inner ear; contains cells sensitive to sound waves

Codominance – the existence of two alleles for a certain characteristic where neither dominates

Collagen – a protein that is found in many tissues, including bone

Connective tissue – any tissue that fills in spaces within the body or connects various parts, e.g. adipose tissue

Cornified layer – a layer of dead cells containing the protein keratin; found on the skin surface

Corpus luteum – a structure within the ovary formed when an ovum is released from a follicle; secretes progesterone

Cristae – folds of the inner membrane of mitochondria on which later stages of anaerobic respiration occur

Cytoplasm – the part of a cell that contains all the cell organelles including the nucleus

DNA (deoxyribonucleic acid) – the molecule that makes up chromosomes and carries the genetic code

Deamination – a reaction taking place in the liver, where amino acids are broken down to carbohydrate and urea

Dermis – the inner layer of the skin

Diaphragm – the muscular sheet that separates the horse's thorax from the abdomen

Diastole – the stage of the heart beat when the heart is relaxed

Diffusion – the movement of particles of a gas or liquid from an area of higher concentration to one of lower concentration

Digestion – enzyme-controlled breakdown of larger molecules in food to smaller ones that may be absorbed

Dipeptide – substance formed when two amino acid molecules join together

Diploid – pertaining to a cell which contains two of each kind of chromosome

Disaccharide – a sugar made up of two monosaccharide molecules joined together

Duodenum – a short part of the small intestine between the stomach and jejunum

Egestion – the excretion of indigestible food from the horse's body

Embryo – an animal as it develops from the fertilised egg

Emulsification – the breaking up of large fat droplets into smaller ones that can disperse in water

Endolymph – the fluid contained within the cochlea

Endoplasmic reticulum – a network of membranes contained within most cells that builds new molecules

Enzymes – protein biological catalysts, made by an animal, that speed up chemical reactions

Epithelium – a tissue that covers many surfaces both inside and outside the body

Expiration – breathing out; the opposite of inspiration

Extensor – a muscle that extends a limb when it contracts

Extracellular – outside of a cell

Faeces – remains of indigestible food, bacteria, mucus, etc., evacuated from the digestive tract

Fertilisation – the joining together of a sperm and egg

Flexor – a muscle that causes a limb to bend when it contracts

Fibrinogen – a blood protein involved in blood clotting

Gamete – sex cell; an egg or sperm cell

Gene – a specific section of DNA that codes for the making of a particular protein

Genome – all the genes in an individual

Genotype – the genes possessed by an animal

Genus – a group of species with similar characteristics

Gestation period – the time between conception and birth

Glomerulus – a network of blood capillaries within the cup of Bowman's capsule in the kidney

Glucagon – a hormone produced by the pancreas in response to low blood sugar levels

Glycogen – a storage polysaccharide made up of long chains of glucose units and stored mainly in the liver and muscles

Glycogenolysis – breakdown of glycogen to glucose

Glycolysis – the first reactions of respiration, where glucose is partly broken down releasing a small amount of energy only

Guanine – one of the four bases of the nucleotides of DNA

Haploid – having only one of each chromosome; the condition of sex cells

Haemoglobin – a red pigment contained within red blood cells that carries oxygen

Hemicellulose – a complex carbohydrate, similar to cellulose, that is found in plant cell walls

Homeostasis – the maintenance of a constant internal environment within a horse's body

Homologous chromosomes – a pair of chromosomes with the same gene sequence and same overall size and shape; found only in the diploid nucleus

Hormone – a chemical that is made in one part of the body and travels via the blood to exert an effect on another; a chemical messenger

Hydrolysis – reaction in which polymers are split by the addition of water; reverse of the condensation reaction

Hydrophilic – describes water-loving molecules, which can therefore mix easily with water

Hydrophobic – describes water-hating molecules, which cannot mix with water

Hypertonic – a solution that is more concentrated (i.e. contains less water) in comparison with another

Hypothalamus – the part of the brain to which the pituitary gland is joined; responsible for many aspects of homeostasis, e.g. control of body temperature

Hypotonic – a solution that is less concentrated (i.e. contains more water) in comparison with another solution

Hypoxia – the condition of low blood oxygen concentration

Ileum – the part of the digestive tract between the duodenum and colon

Immunity – the presence of antibodies effective against a particular disease

Incisor – a tooth at the front of the horse's mouth used for biting off pieces of food for chewing

Ingestion – taking food into the digestive tract

Insoluble – unable to dissolve in water

Insulin – a hormone produced by the pancreas in response to high sugar concentrations in the blood

Intracellular – inside cells

Intrinsic protein – a protein molecule that spans the width of a phospholipid membrane such as the cell membrane

Islets of Langerhans – patches of cells within the horse's pancreas that secrete the hormone insulin

Isomers – molecules with the same molecular formula but with a different structure, i.e. containing the same atoms arranged in different ways

Isotonic – a solution that has the same concentration of water molecules as another

Keratin – the protein that makes up hair and hoof horn

Krebs cycle – Following on from glycolysis, the Krebs cycle takes place in the mitochondria during aerobic respiration

Lacteal – a branch of a lymph vessel found in the centre of a villus of the small intestine

Lactic acid – a chemical produced by horses during anaerobic respiration

Lipase – an enzyme that digests fats

Lumen – space within a tube, such as the cavity of a blood vessel

Lymph node – a part of the lymphatic system that contains large numbers of white blood cells

Lysosome – vesicle produced by the Golgi body containing digestive enzymes

Malphigian layer – a layer of cells at the base of the epidermis which divides to form new cells which contain the pigment melanin

Meiosis – cell division where homologous chromosomes separate, producing four haploid cells from one diploid cell; the form of cell division that produces the sex cells

Meninges – membranes surrounding the brain and spinal cord

Metabolism – all the chemical reactions that take place within the horse's body

Mitochondrion – a cell organelle that is the power house of the cell, producing energy from respiration

Mitosis – a type of cell division that results in two identical daughter cells formed from one parent cell

Molar – a large flattened tooth for grinding, found at the back of the horse's mouth

Monosaccharide – a carbohydrate composed of a single sugar molecule, e.g. glucose or maltose

Mucosa – the inner layer of the digestive-tract wall

Mutation – an unpredictable change in the chromosome make-up of an animal

Natural selection – the process by which only the fittest and strongest organisms survive to reproduce within an environment

Nephron – a kidney tubule where urine is formed before being excreted

Nerve – a group of nerve fibres surrounded by connective tissue

Oesophagus – a tubular part of the digestive tract between the throat and the stomach

Organelle – an area in a cell that carries out a particular function

Osmosis – the movement of water molecules through a partially permeable membrane from a region of higher concentration to one of lower concentration

Ovulation – the release of an egg from an ovary

Oxygen deficit – the amount of oxygen needed following exercise to convert the lactic acid produced during the exercise to glycogen

Oxyhaemoglobin – a molecule of haemoglobin that has combined with oxygen

Partially permeable membrane – a membrane that allows only some substances to pass through

Pathogen – an organism that causes disease

Pectin – soluble polysaccharide found in plant cell walls

Peptide bond – the link between two amino acids

Permeable – allowing substances to pass through

Phenotype – the actual characteristics displayed by an organism resulting from its genotype and environment

Placenta – the organ by which the foetus is connected, in the uterus, to the dam

Polypeptide – a substance that is made from large numbers of amino acids in a chain

Polysaccharide – a polymer molecule made by joining many single mono-saccharides (monomers) together

Protease – an enzyme that digests protein

Protein – a polymer molecule made by joining many amino acids together

Receptor – part of the horse's body that receives stimuli

Reflex action – an automatic response to a stimulus

Respiration – the release of energy from carbohydrates that occurs in all living cells within the horse's body

Ribosome – a cell organelle that makes proteins

Semilunar valve – prevents backflow of blood from an artery into the ventricle of the heart

Serum – blood plasma that has had the clotting protein fibrinogen removed

Solute – a substance that dissolves in water, or another solvent, to make a solution

Solvent – a substance in which other substances dissolve

Sphincter – a muscle around a tube that closes it by contracting

Starch – the polysaccharide storage material of plants, made from hundreds of glucose molecules linked together

Sucrose – a non-reducing disaccharide sugar

Synovial joint – a joint between two bones allowing free movement

Systole – contraction of the heart muscle

Testis – male reproductive organ that produces the male gametes or sperm

Thorax – the chest

Tissue – a group of similar cells that together fulfil a particular function

Tissue fluid – fluid derived from blood plasma that bathes tissue cells

Toxin – a poison; often produced by pathogens within the body

Trachea – a semi-rigid tube that carries air from the throat to the bronchi

Urine – a watery fluid containing urea and other excretory products; excreted by the kidney

Uterus (womb) – muscular organ with a soft lining for carrying the foetus during pregnancy

Vein – a blood vessel that returns blood to the heart

Vena cava – the main vein returning deoxygenated blood collected from the body to the right atrium of the heart

Ventricle – one of the two lower chambers of the heart

Zygote – the cell formed when the two gametes (egg and sperm) fuse at fertilisation

Index